THE
PREGNANCY
SURVIVAL MANUAL

THE
PREGNANCY
SURVIVAL MANUAL

Geoffrey Chamberlain MD., FRCS., FRCOG.
Professor of Obstetrics and Gynaecology, St George's Hospital Medical School

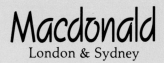

Macdonald
London & Sydney

A QED BOOK

Published by Macdonald & Co (Publishers) Ltd
Maxwell House
Worship Street
London

First published 1984
ISBN 0 356 10424-9

Chamberlain, Geoffrey, 1930-
   The Pregnancy Survival Manual
   1. Pregnancy 2. Childbirth
   I. Title
   618.2   RG524

ISBN 0-356-10424-9

Typeset in Great Britain by QV Typesetting Limited
Printed in Hong Kong by Lee Fung Asco Limited
Origination by Hong Kong Graphics Arts Services Centre

All statements in this book giving information or advice
are believed to be true and accurate at the time of going to
press but neither the author nor the publishers can
accept any legal liability for errors or omissions.

This book was designed and produced by
QED Publishing Limited
32 Kingly Court, London W1

Senior Editor: Jim Miles
Editor: Liz Davies
Design: Graham Davis Associates
Art Editor: Graham Davis
Designer: Kevin Ryan
Editorial Director: Christopher Fagg
*Art Director:*Alastair Campbell

Photographs
Daisy Hayes
John Heseltine
Ian Howes
Richard and Sally Greenhill
Sarah King
John Larsson (St George's Medical School)
Special thanks to Dr Peter Flute and
Dr Rashmi Varma

Illustrations
Craig Austin
Bob Chapman
Edwina Keene
Mark Taylor
Paula Youens

The author and publishers gratefully
acknowledge the mothers and fathers
and their babies who helped to make
this book possible, together with the
midwifery and medical staff of
St George's Hospital, Tooting, London

FOREWORD

For some time now there has been a fashion for decrying the expert obstetrician. There are people who consider themselves 'radical' who maintain that childbirth should be taken out of the hands of the hospital-based obstetrician and given back to Nature. If their advice is followed to the letter there is a very real risk that Nature will do as she usually does and waste a great deal of life.

Which is why I for one believe we very much need our obstetricians with their vast stores of knowledge and experience to take care of us as we make the interesting but potentially hazardous journey through a pregnancy and a birth. A good deal can be left to Nature (and of course every good obstetrician knows that and uses the body's own reserves and abilities to aid his efforts to care for a mother and her child) but more is needed. And this books tells every mother just what that 'more' is.

Professor Chamberlain brings to his text not just a great gift for organization of a complex subject (you can find what you need to know very quickly in these beautifully laid out pages), but also a real affection for mothers and babies. Every word shows that he cares for his patients as people, not just as containers of babies which have to be extracted, but at the same time it is clear that he is a superb technician, well able to advise on how to cope with the sort of problems that may arise even in the most natural of processes. This is a book that, though designed to inform and reassure mothers, could teach a good deal to some other workers in the field of obstetrics. Including those who want to exclude obstetricians from childbirth!

It is above all a reliable book. The facts that are here presented are as accurate as they can possibly be. The ideas that are discussed are dealt with honestly. This is a book mothers can trust. With its help they can travel through their pregnancies with peace of mind and understanding of what is happening to them.

I congratulate Professor Chamberlain for his book — and I congratulate any woman who has personal cause to read it. Enjoy your pregnancy, and your baby!

CLAIRE RAYNER

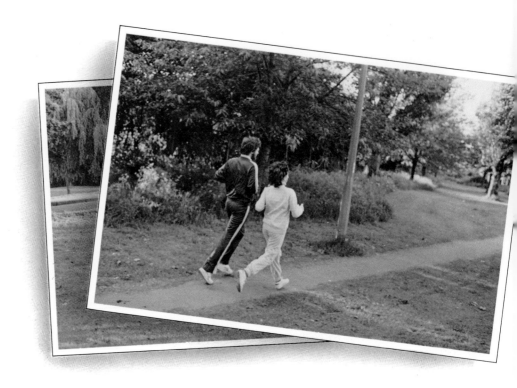

PRE-PREGNANCY CARE

For many women today, pregnancy is the result of a conscious decision to have a baby and is not something forced on them by poverty, ignorance or demanding husbands. Naturally, you will want to ensure that you are in the best possible health to face what will be a physically demanding experience. If you look after yourself in the weeks and months before you become pregnant, your body will be in a good position to help the rapidly growing embryo in the early period of pregnancy, before you are even aware of it and before you begin your formal antenatal care.

CONTRACEPTION

You have decided that you want to have a baby. The first thing that must happen, of course, is that you must stop whatever form of contraception you have been using. If you have an intrauterine device (IUD) you will need to seek the help of your family planning clinic or GP to have it removed. You should do this a couple of months before you start trying to conceive.

Similarly, if you have been taking oral contraceptives you will need to plan ahead to stop at least two cycles before trying to conceive. (You could use a mechanical form of contraceptive such as the sheath plus spermicide in the meantime.) The pill consists of one or two hormones (depending on the type of pill taken) which affect the body by interfering with egg-release and the union of the egg with sperm. The effects of these hormones are known to remain in the body for some time.

Mechanical contraceptive methods such as the sheath, the cap or the diaphragm have little general effect on the body and so do not need to be stopped in advance.

Accidental conception

Conversely, some babies are conceived while couples are still using contraceptives. If this happens after failure of one of the barrier methods (cap, sheath, diaphragm) there are no serious implications for the embryo. Should you become pregnant even though you have an IUD still in the uterus you must consult your family doctor as soon as possible. At first the growing embryo does not fill the uterus and the IUD can be removed without much problem. Once 12 to 14 weeks have passed, however, the removal might cause difficulty and you may be counselled to keep it in place. It will do no harm to the growing baby and the device can be delivered after the baby is born. If you conceive following a failure of the pill, stop taking it and consult your doctor or family planning clinic.

THE WAY WE LIVE

Nutrition

In other species, the female tends to boost her diet and to achieve a good level of fitness before conceiving. It is not considered necessary for women in developed countries to prepare themselves in this way but, instinctively, some women still find themselves eating more when they are trying to conceive.

Most women in the West who have a varied diet will get enough protein (body-building foods), carbohydrates (calorie- and energy-providing foods) and a sufficiency of vitamins and minerals. Recently, there has been discussion about the value of giving vitamin supplements to women who have had babies with abnormalities of the nervous system, such as spina bifida. The evidence so far, however, is inconclusive.

Since most of us eat without thinking too much about our diet, eating those things we like or can afford, it may help you to know something about the theory of nutrition. Theoretically, food is needed for three reasons:
1 To supply material for growth and repair; this comes from proteins which are particularly necessary in pregnancy to supply the growing body of the fetus inside the mother.
2 To provide fuel to keep the body working; this comes from fats and carbohydrates. We take these when we are hungry and they stock us up for the next few hours.
3 To process the chemical actions in the body; these actions involve minerals and vitamins which come as incidentals in our food. We do not notice them, but they are essential, particularly in pregnancy, when many vitamins are needed to help the growth of the unborn child.

Proteins, used for repairing and building tissues, may come from animal or vegetable sources. Meat is about 20 per cent protein and bread 10 per cent, while some beans and pulses contain an even higher proportion. The body needs about 40 g of protein a day, best obtained in mixed fashion. Protein is made up of individual molecules of amino acids which occur in different proportions in different forms. The body's digestive system breaks down into much smaller units all proteins eaten and the individual amino acids are then reconstituted in new ways inside the body. Many are essential for growth.

In pregnancy, the growing fetus and uterus require much more protein than does the stable adult body. If dietary protein is lacking in some of the amino acid constituents, the mother breaks down her own protein tissues in the muscles to provide the fetus with his needs. In this sense, the fetus is a parasite on the mother and will usually get enough protein; it will be the mother who suffers if she does not take enough in her diet.

Fuel

The energy requirements of food can be measured in calories, a unit which measures the amount of heat a food is capable of providing. Most people eat a diet containing about 2,000 calories a day, although someone doing hard manual work might need up to 4,000. In pregnancy, a diet of between 2,500 and 3,000 calories is probably about right. If you take more calories than that, you do not help your baby any more, you merely put on weight. Most of the calories we take in are used to maintain our body's actions — the muscles that hold us up, those with which we walk and breathe, the heart's action and the activity of the gut in digesting food; these all require energy which comes from calories, mostly derived from carbohydrates and fats. Carbohydrates make up between 50 and 60 per cent of the food we eat, for as well as the obvious carbohydrates, such as sugar, there are starches and celluloses in food. Sugar comes in the sweet things (biscuits, cakes and confectionery) and some add it to drinks of coffee and tea. Starch is found in bulky vegetables such as potatoes, wheat and rice. Some of this bulk is broken down in the body to make sugar. Cellulose is not digested by human beings (although other animals can use it). It forms the bulk of the food and passes undigested through the body and out in the faeces.

The body gets its fuel from many sources. Most of us take our fuel in the form of carbohydrate, but fats are a more efficient source of fuel.

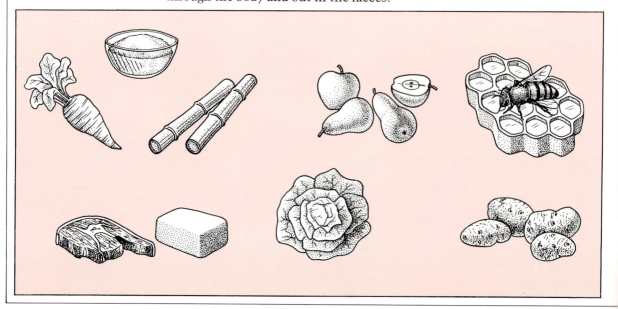

Fats are important in food, not just for their calories, but because they improve the taste of food and because some vitamins such as vitamin D are only soluble in fat. Generally, we get our fat from meat- and animal-derived products, such as milk, butter and cheese. In meat, there is the obvious fat around the outside of the cut, just under the animal's skin, and fat cells also tucked between the muscle cells which we do not notice. Fat is an efficient source of energy, providing twice the energy derived from the same weight of carbohydrates. If you are on a low-carbohydrate diet, you should remember that a slice of bread with a thin smear of butter or margarine can contain as many calories in the margarine as in the bread.

Vitamins are needed in minute amounts only. Their nomenclature is haphazard; they were named alphabetically as they were discovered and, in some cases, they are sub-classified by means of suffix numbers, for example the B group of vitamins. Vitamins take no part in providing energy or building materials in the body but catalyze the chemical processes that go on. They might be compared to oil needed for an engine; the oil itself is not an energy source, but lubricates the pistons so that the engine works; without it the engine would seize up. Excessive deficiency of vitamins leads to well known diseases like rickets (lack of vitamin D) and scurvy (lack of vitamin C). These are rare in the West, but mild deficiency can occur, particularly among pregnant women. Many of us take only just sufficient vitamins in our daily food; the same diet is insufficient to provide for both mother and fetus. The growing fetus demands many more vitamins than his mother, so you should pay particular attention to the level of vitamins in your diet. Paradoxically, there is no value in taking more vitamins than mother and baby need; vitamins are absorbed from the intestine only according to the needs of the body and any extra is excreted. In pregnancy, there is usually no need to take large amounts of extra vitamins in the form of tablets. Folic acid, however, is needed in pregnancy in larger amounts than most diets provide; antenatal clinics provide most women with folic acid tablets.

The body also needs minerals. These are the basic elements of chemistry and minute amounts of them are needed to keep body processes going. For instance, iron (which comes from meat) is needed to make haemoglobin, the blood pigment that travels around the body carrying oxygen in the red blood cells. The actions of muscles require calcium and magnesium; those of the thyroid gland, iodine. Generally speaking, diet in Western countries is adequate in these minerals. In pregnancy, iron requirements are increased enormously, for the baby needs this mineral to build his own blood and muscles. It is probably wise to supplement the content of the pregnant woman's diet with iron and this, too, is given in most antenatal clinics.

Exercise

Some years ago I would have begun this section by complaining that most people did not take enough exercise. Nowadays, with the popularizing of jogging and aerobics, and the emergence of countless gyms and health clubs, it is becoming increasingly unfashionable to be unfit. This can only be an advantage to women approaching pregnancy, for they will be in a better position to cope with the physical demands of pregnancy and childbirth.

You may, of course, be concerned about the level of activity that you can safely continue in pregnancy. Generally speaking, any activity which you have been following regularly prior to pregnancy, can be safely continued providing you feel confident about it — and your increasing bulk will allow it. Some particularly exerting or hazardous activities such as skiing, horse-riding, skin-diving or motor racing would not be advisable, as common sense would suggest.

If you have not embarked on a keep-fit programme of one sort or another then a little gentle exercise such as walking a mile or so each day or swimming twice a week would be very beneficial. In later pregnancy many women find swimming very relaxing — it literally gets the weight off their feet.

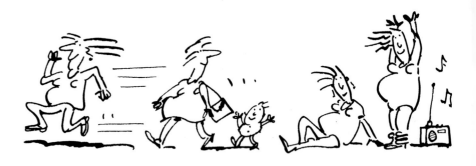

Work

Many women have dual responsibilities for work within the home and in formal paid employment outside it. Once you become pregnant, these responsibilities can become a burden. Although the growing embryo is very small, the effects on your body and on your emotions are enormous, even from the first weeks. It is not at all unusual to feel extremely weary during the first few months. You will have to consider your business, domestic and social obligations and try to find ways of sparing yourself.

Your job may involve specific hazards for the growing embryo. If you work, for example, in the chemical or cleaning industries you will be in contact with powerful chemicals which you should avoid when pregnant. Another obvious hazard is the use of X-rays; this is a problem not just in hospitals but in industries where they are used to check the strength of metal objects, and in the security business where they are used to look inside parcels. Pesticides and insecticides are all highly toxic substances and women may handle them in production or in horticulture. Certain chemicals used in dyeing, hairdressing and dry cleaning also have side effects on the mother and the unborn child. The hazards listed above are fairly obvious; of less proven harm are solvents such as those found in petrol and paint. If you have any doubts about substances that you work with, contact your Health and Safety Officer at work, or your trade union. If your job involves lifting heavy weights or simply standing for long periods of time, you should obviously not continue with this aspect of your duties and you should discuss this with your employer.

All work requires effort and it is probable that the more fatiguing jobs can have some effect on your unborn child. Hard physical work can be associated with a higher incidence of early pre-term labour and smaller babies. If your work is outside the home, even getting to work can be a problem. Public

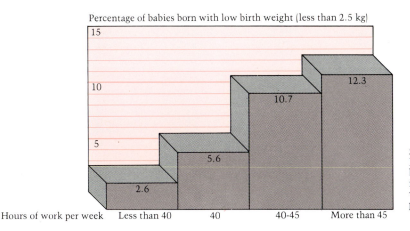

Percentage of babies born with low birth weight (less than 2.5 kg)

Hours of work per week | Less than 40 — 2.6 | 40 — 5.6 | 40-45 — 10.7 | More than 45 — 12.3

Statistically, you are more likely to have a pre-term baby of lower birth weight if you do hard physical work during your pregnancy.

transport, with its smoky, tiring and stressful atmosphere, is not the best place for women to be in early pregnancy and taking your own transport can be even more stressful.

However, it would be quite wrong to suggest that, ideally, a pregnant woman should abandon her job and devote herself to contemplation of her expanding body. Boredom and frustration can have just as harmful effects as over-exertion. For many, economic forces will impose pressure on the woman to continue working for as long as possible. For others there is the dilemma that the childbearing years often coincide with a time that is critical to career advancement. Happily, legislation now makes it possible for some women to take time off to have their babies without losing their position. Although this by no means solves all the problems it has clearly been a welcome development.

YOUR RIGHTS AT WORK

All women are entitled to time off work for antenatal care, without loss of pay. If your condition means that you are no longer capable of carrying out your duties, you should be offered an alternative job, if there is one available.

Maternity pay and maternity leave
To qualify for these you must have worked for the same employer full-time (more than 16 hours per week) for at least two years, or part-time (8 to 16 hours) for five years by the 11th week before the baby is due.
and
You must work up to the 11th week (although you may work longer).

Maternity pay is paid for six weeks at the rate of 9/10ths of your basic pay, less the amount received in maternity allowance.

Maternity leave can begin from 11 weeks before the baby is due, and lasts for up to 29 weeks after the birth.

To secure your rights you must inform your employer, in writing, at least three weeks before you leave:
● that you are leaving to have a baby;
● the expected date of the birth
● that you intend to exercise your right to return to the job.

Many women continue working well into their pregnancy. If you enjoy it and your health remains good, there is no reason to give it up.

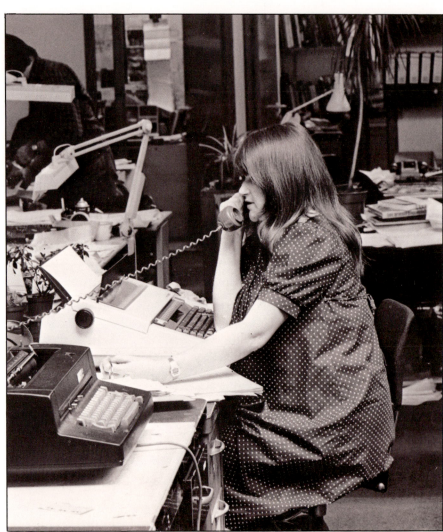

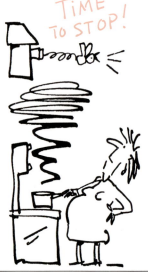

The whole problem of work in pregnancy is a difficult one. If the work you do is not fatiguing, does not involve hazardous chemicals or radiation, and you are used to it, then it is probably wise to continue. You will be bored sitting at home doing nothing and work can be a stimulating place, where you can talk to your colleagues and think about your future. If, however, your work is fatiguing or the effort of getting to work is overtiring, you should seriously consider giving it up. There are no hard and fast rules about this, except for those in jobs that involve specific chemical or physical hazards. There are many issues to consider and you must decide what will be right for your particular circumstances.

AVOIDABLE RISKS

Many health problems are self-induced. They can arise from abuse of alcohol, tobacco and other drugs and these can all contribute to problems in pregnancy. If you have a problem with any of these and you are serious about giving your child the best start in life then it is important to consider them before your conceive.

Tobacco

The inhalation of tobacco has a retarding effect on the growth of the fetus and the more the mother smokes the greater the effect. Women who stop smoking and who avoid smoky environments have a much better chance of producing a healthy well-developed baby. Unfortunately, it is not known exactly which of the influences of cigarette smoking affect the unborn child. Obviously, while the mother is inhaling cigarette smoke she is not inhaling oxygen and this in turn cuts down the oxygen supply to the fetus. Cigarette smoke contains carbon monoxide, and this may affect the blood of the growing child. The nicotine and tar products from cigarettes are also implicated but, as they are not the sole problem, it does little good just to switch to a lower-tar brand.

Giving up smoking

The most important factor is to want to stop. Consider the advantages of not smoking on your own health and that of the unborn baby. Remember that although the benefits of stopping will not show in your health for a few years, they will be apparent almost immediately in the baby. Be realistic and face up to the fact that eventually you will find other pleasures and other ways of relaxing.

You have made the decision, now comes the stopping. Most people find it easier to succeed if they stop completely rather than cutting down gradually. Try to find a time in the next week or two, when you are comparatively free of stress and then, with the help of your partner, stop. Chewing gum may be helpful, or going through the ritual of making a cup of tea or coffee may ease the difficulty. Some people try going for a brisk walk in the fresh air, while others go for a drive. You could try doing an energetic job in the house, take a bath or just clean your teeth. The important thing is to have some alternative action, so make a list and keep it to hand.

Talk about it with your doctor if it is particularly difficult. He may recommend some more formal help. He can prescribe a nicotine-containing chewing gum (Nicorette) to provide you with a small amount of the stimulant drug from tobacco. This will not have as bad an effect on the fetus as smoking and it may serve to help you over the first month. You can buy dummy cigarettes or filters to reduce the amount of smoke that goes into your mouth. These are a help to some but the major factor will be your motivation.

Doctors can prescribe tablets which make cigarettes taste nasty. There are courses in formal acupuncture, psychotherapy and hypnosis. Details can be obtained from your doctor but few people who smoke actually have to resort to this. An extreme form of treatment is aversion therapy: every time a cigarette is taken an unpleasant stimulus (such as an electric shock) accompanies it; this should be avoided in pregnancy.

To stop smoking *is* difficult. It requires concentration and determination from you and your partner. It will help if your partner stops smoking at the same time as you and he may be persuaded to do so if he considers the dangers of passive smoking. Cigarettes affect not only those who smoke them but also those who live in an atmosphere polluted by cigarette smoke. For this reason a prospective father who smokes will be having an effect on the mother-to-be at a secondary level and, at a third level, the growing embryo itself.

Even if *you* do not smoke, you can be affected by a smoker sitting next to you.

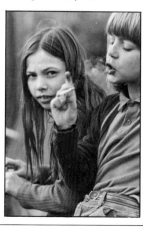

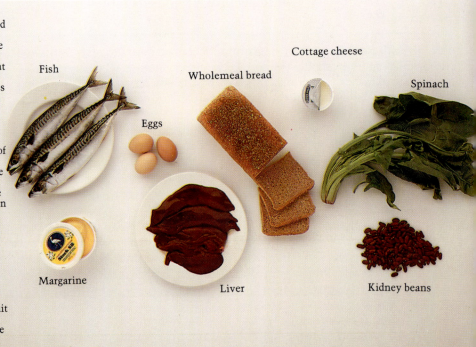

Pregnant women need more protein, vitamins and minerals than usual to allow for fetal growth. The best guide is to cut down the amount of sugar and fat and step up the amount of fresh fruit, fresh vegetables and cereals. Iron (found in liver and spinach) is especially important. It is part of the haemoglobin molecule and is therefore involved in the transport of oxygen to all organs, tissues and cells. Since the body does not store sufficient iron to meet the needs of pregnancy, an iron supplement is usually recommended. Calcium, found in milk, cheese and yogurt, is also important for fetal development. At least 300g (half a pint) of milk shoud be taken each day. Protein is found in lean meat, fish, eggs, cheese and nuts. Fresh fruit and vegetables contain vitamin C which helps the body to absorb iron. Folic

Fish

Eggs

Wholemeal bread

Cottage cheese

Spinach

Margarine

Liver

Kidney beans

Alcohol

Alcohol is a pleasant relaxant widely used in the West. Many people enjoy an occasional drink to oil the wheels of social behaviour. However, it is also a poison which affects growing cells. In early pregnancy the baby's cells are growing very rapidly and it would be wise not to drink alcohol at all during this period. If this is too difficult you should cut down and restrict yourself to a couple of glasses of wine on special occasions. Although this is better than carrying on at the same level, it must be stressed that there is no safe lower limit of alcohol before or during pregnancy.

Giving up alcohol

The most important step towards giving up alcohol during pregnancy is to believe that it may have some effect on your baby. There is no safe amount of alcohol that can be taken in pregnancy, even the smallest doses go across to the developing embryo and fetus. In considering this problem you must weigh up, on the one hand, the pleasure you get from the drink and the way it helps to reduce tension with, on the other hand, the advantage your child will derive from being spared these poisons. Remember too that you do not have to give up all alcohol for ever.

The most important factor is to want to give up. Once you have decided to stop, do so at a time when you think there is going to be relatively little stress for a week or two. If you can, avoid social groups that go to the pub after work (or, worse still, at lunchtime) and then press you to have a drink. If you have to be with them, drink something that is non-alcoholic but looks sociable such as tonic water with ice and lemon or a glass of apple juice. The easiest way not to drink with a crowd is to leave your glass two-thirds full, then when the next round comes you can pass without a fuss.

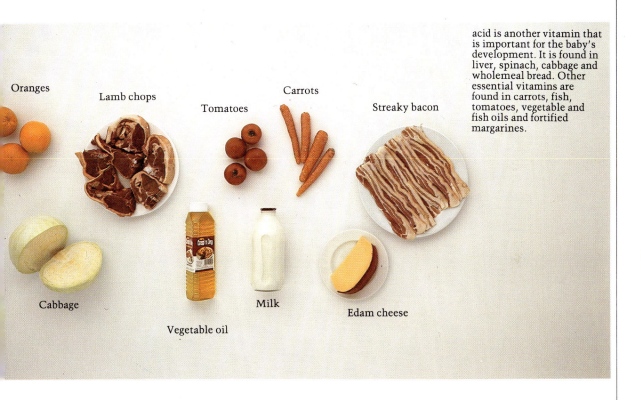

Oranges

Lamb chops

Tomatoes

Carrots

Streaky bacon

Cabbage

Vegetable oil

Milk

Edam cheese

acid is another vitamin that is important for the baby's development. It is found in liver, spinach, cabbage and wholemeal bread. Other essential vitamins are found in carrots, fish, tomatoes, vegetable and fish oils and fortified margarines.

If you are used to taking alcohol at home the easiest way to reduce the habit is not to keep any alcohol in the house. If there is no bottle of sherry in the cupboard, you cannot turn to it at lunchtime when the world is black. Talk about this freely with your partner and try to persuade him to give up also during your pregnancy, so that together you can grow a healthy child.

More formal methods of cutting down alcohol are rarely needed by the pregnant woman. Nature often lends a hand so that chemical changes take place which may make alcohol taste unpleasant. This happens most often during the critical early months. Psychological and drug treatments do exist where the patient is given a drug to make the taking of any alcohol most unpleasant; vomiting and severe headaches result and such therapy should not be undertaken in pregnancy.

Other drugs of addiction

The stronger drugs of addiction have dramatic effects on the unborn child in the earliest days. Heroin, hashish, marijuana and LSD are all harmful to the young embryo and should be stopped *before* pregnancy. Sometimes women who take these drugs have difficulty in stopping and further advice should be sought from their doctor. As well as being harmful to their total health they are extremely harmful to the unborn child.

Some drugs that may affect the fetus

It is very important to consider carefully the use of *any* drugs or medicines both immediately prior to and then throughout your pregnancy. Some women are on long term treatments for conditions they have had for years, such as asthma. It is as important to discuss this with your doctor as any new drugs. When you take a drug during pregnancy some part of it will almost certainly cross the placenta to the fetus; this depends upon the chemical properties of the drug, and the following pages deal with some of these drugs and their possible side-effects.

Antibiotics	All antibiotics cross the placenta and most are perfectly safe to the fetus. Those in the penicillin group, for example, have no untoward effect on the unborn child. However, some sulphonimides can affect the capacity in the fetus's blood of protein binding to the naturally produced bilirubin and so the newborn baby may be jaundiced. Tetracyclin attaches itself to bone, causing yellow discolouration and slight limitation in the growth activity. The alteration of colour does not matter, for most bone is hidden, but there is one place where specialized bone is seen — the teeth. It causes a yellow-brown discolouration of the milk teeth and a weakness of the enamel so that caries is more likely to follow. It does not affect the permanent dentition that follows later in life; tetracyclin is probably best avoided in pregnancy. Streptomycin, used for more severe infections and for tuberculosis, may affect the child's hearing in some of the higher frequency ranges although it does not seem to alter hearing at speaking range. These side effects are well known and your doctor will be very careful when prescribing an antibiotic for you in pregnancy. Consider also that if you decide not to take antibiotics when they have been prescribed for you, you risk exposing the unborn child to the effects of a severe infection which may be more harmful than the potential hazards of some of these antibiotics.
Aspirin	This simple analgesic has been blamed for producing abnormalities. Research is based upon animal work where very high dosages were used in a ratio many times greater than that which a woman would take in pregnancy. There is no real evidence that aspirin causes abnormalities if taken in moderation.
Anti-vomiting drugs	Some of the anti-vomiting drugs have been blamed for abnormalities. The evidence for this is thin. Vomiting occurs among two-thirds of women in pregnancy and it may be that the more severe aspects of this could be of greater harm to the developing embryo than the drugs used to stop it. Variations of your internal metabolism may be associated with deformity and we do not know the full effects of this on the developing tissues. Several drugs have been suspected and some have been the subject of court cases but a court of law is not the place to settle scientific alternatives. Ask your doctor's advice and he will give you a drug which will be safe for you if the degree of vomiting warrants it. Remember, too, that most doctors are conservative when prescribing drugs and they are especially conservative when prescribing for a pregnant woman.
Hormones	Progesterone is a hormone which is made naturally in the placenta. Sometimes it is necessary to give artificial progesterone to a woman to make up for a lack of the natural product. There is a slight risk that certain progesterone preparations can produce minor alterations so that a female embryo might develop external signs of masculinity. Correction is a minor thing but there could be psychological upset. If progesterone has to be given in early pregnancy there are some preparations available which are safer than others.

Cortisone may be used in various forms for the treatment of long-term conditions such as ulcerative colitis or lupus erythematosis. If a woman is already taking such drugs she may have to continue them into pregnancy in order to stay well. Despite several reports, there is no solid evidence that cortisone in ordinary dosage, taken by a woman who requires it, causes an effect to the fetus. Should you be taking such a drug and discover you are pregnant, talk with your doctor before stopping a steroid; the effects on the embryo of any flare-up of the condition for which you are taking the cortisone may be worse than those of the drug itself.

Over 400 drugs have been alleged to affect other species but probably fewer than a dozen have a serious effect in the human. The developing embryo is tough. When you consider the large amount of chemicals, food additives and medicines that most women take in pregnancy, very few babies are actually affected. Drug-produced abnormalities are rare and proper consultation at your clinic with your doctor will ensure that you carry your baby safely.

Drugs in perspective

FIXED RISKS

Pregnancy occurs in young women, most of whom are fit and well. They are no more at risk from general diseases than any other group of the population, but a small number of women enter pregnancy with an existing medical condition which is being properly cared for by the family doctor, possibly with the help of a hospital consultant. Forty years ago many women like this were told not to get pregnant because it was feared that the illness would affect the pregnancy and that pregnancy would exacerbate the condition. Now, with better knowledge of medicine, many doctors are not giving such restrictive advice. Women with all sorts of chronic medical conditions which previously would have made pregnancy inadvisable are now producing perfectly healthy and normal children.

Diabetes is a disorder which affects up to one per cent of the population in the reproductive age group. The condition is caused by an inability of the body to control the level of blood sugar derived from the carbohydrates in food. Some diabetics have to take regular amounts of the hormone insulin, to deal with the problem. Provided they know about this beforehand and their medical advisers keep a close watch, most diabetics continue through pregnancy and produce a normal child without problems. Especially careful monitoring is needed, however, for the mother can have wider swings in her insulin requirements during pregnancy than beforehand. Diabetic mothers have a slight increase in the risk of pre-eclampsia; the baby often grows larger and comes out bigger than from a woman who has not got diabetes. This too can be controlled to some extent by careful regulation of the diabetic process.

Diabetes

For these reasons, the diabetic woman often needs closer surveillance in pregnancy and may be asked to come into hospital during the antenatal period, even though she is feeling perfectly well. This is to provide extra care in balancing her insulin requirements and to watch the fetus more closely. She will probably be induced before term and may require a Caesarian section. Following delivery, the diabetic mother will require careful watching but after a week or two she will return home just as she was before pregnancy.

Heart disease	Most heart disease in young people follows rheumatic fever. With the improvement in living conditions and the widespread use of antibiotics, this is now a less frequent and a much less severe condition in the young. Any woman who has heart disease is putting an extra load on her heart by having a pregnancy, but this can be controlled provided she and her doctors take extra care during the pregnancy and delivery. More bed rest will be required, some of which may have to be in hospital. Minor infections which may not affect any other woman could be serious to a woman with heart disease and so antibiotics may be prescribed more frequently, for example to cover times like removal of teeth or to deal with a bad cold. Delivery requires special skills to remove all but the minimum load to the woman and, after delivery, the care of the child requires careful planning, for the work of a mother with heart disease should be limited.
Hypertension	Chronically raised blood pressure is unusual in the age group of mothers having babies. When it does occur it must be watched carefully, for it may get sharply worse in pregnancy. The woman must be prepared to spend some extra time in hospital but she can look forward to a normal baby and no worsening of her condition during her pregnancy.
Chronic urinary infection	This used to be another bar to pregnancy but, with sensible antibiotic regimes now established, most women with chronic urinary infection can go through pregnancy normally. There is a small risk of hypertension but this is watched for in the antenatal clinic.
Chronic skin diseases	Many women who get pregnant have psoriasis or chronic erythema. These conditions are sometimes slightly improved in pregnancy because of the increased steriods circulating in the blood. In themselves, they are no bar to a healthy pregnancy.
Venereal diseases (Sexually transmitted diseases)	These may be acquired at the same time as pregnancy starts. They should be diagnosed and treated energetically in early pregnancy for, if cured, there is no reason why the fetus should be affected. It would be dangerous, however, to deliver a fetus through an area in which there was an active gonorrhea or herpes infection. If a woman has any doubts about these she should talk urgently to her own GP or the doctor at the antenatal clinic to get the appropriate tests performed and treatment started.
Cancer	Few women in the age group of pregnancy have cancer. Unfortunately, the treatment of cancer can affect the unborn child, for example, irradiation or some of the drugs used to kill the actively growing cells. Cancer itself does not cause any abnormalities to the unborn child, nor do cancer cells cross the placenta, but the treatments for them may do so and this should be discussed urgently with the doctor in the antenatal clinic. These illnesses are usually known about before pregnancy starts. The guidance of the doctors in pregnancy will be modified by their knowledge of these conditions but in nearly every case the woman will produce a normal healthy baby and will not herself be affected by the pregnancy.

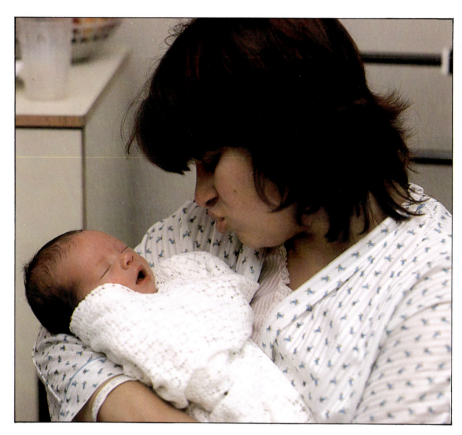

The vast majority of mothers have happy pregnancies and produce healthy babies. The fears of producing a child with any abnormality are, happily, usually groundless.

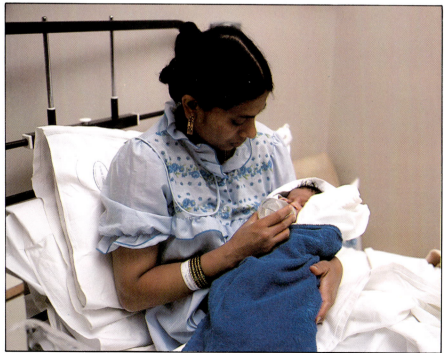

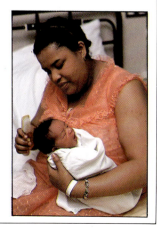

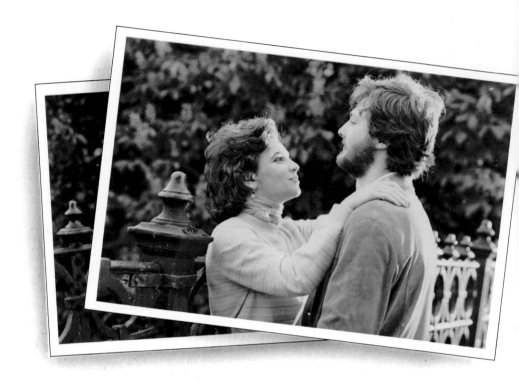

CONCEPTION

Many couples wish to express their feelings for one another and their commitment to their relationship by producing children. Of course, this is a completely individual decision and you will have to consider how many children you would like and at what intervals to have them. Happily, modern methods of contraception give you the opportunity to regulate nature to a large extent so that your plans can be carried out (see Chapter 9). However, for some, it is not easy to start a pregnancy, while for others pregnancy seems to happen all too easily. To understand why this is so, it is necessary to go back a little into the normal reproductive life of a woman.

HOW A WOMAN CONCEIVES

The eggs

When a girl is born, each of her two ovaries contains over 250,000 potential eggs. This is greatly in excess of what she will need and it means that the ovaries are stuffed with potential babies. During infancy and early childhood, these cells do not alter very much, but just about the time of puberty they start to develop.

Most girls start menstruating between the ages of 11 and 13. Within a year of this the hormone changes which accompany menstruation start to act on the primitive egg cells. By the age of 14 or 15, a small number of eggs start to develop with each menstrual cycle. In the early days of the cycle, between 50 and 100 potential eggs start to swell and move towards the surface. On about Day 12 of a normal cycle, one egg swells very much more than the others. This follicle grows to about the size of a woman's thumbnail. It is filled with fluid under tension and contains the almost-ready egg—the one that is going to burst in this particular menstrual cycle.

On each side of the uterus is a tubular structure (the Fallopian tubes) which services the ovaries, rather like a petrol pump hose services cars in a garage. Just before the follicle containing the egg (ovum) is due to mature, one of the tubes moves in the direction of the ovary. The end of the tube is surrounded by a series of finger-like appendages rather like an open sea anemone under water. These embrace the developing follicle and the finger-like growths hang on to the sides of the ovary. On Day 14, the follicle bursts and the primitive egg is taken straight into the Fallopian tube. The egg, with its surrounding cells, now lies in the outer end of the Fallopian tube. It is a passive object, about the size of the point of a pin, with no power of movement.

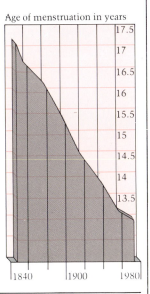

Age of menstruation in years

17.5
17
16.5
16
15.5
15
14.5
14
13.5

1840   1900   1980

The sperm

At intercourse, the man deposits semen in the upper part of the vagina. On average each ejaculation consists of 200,000,000 sperm, but only a very small number of them are in contact with the neck of the womb (the cervix). The most active of these pass up through the cervical canal towards the mucus plug which blocks the canal. If the woman is not within 24 hours of ovulation, the mucus molecules in this plug are higgledy-piggledy and prevent most sperm from passing through. However, within 12 hours of ovulation the molecules straighten out and allow the sperm to travel. Rather like swimmers in an Olympic pool, they race up the cervical canal and travel in the fluid lining the uterus. The earlier part of this journey is across the uterus, where the sperm travel in a haphazard fashion. Some arrive by chance at the upper end of the uterus and pass into the Fallopian tubes on each side. Obviously those that go into the Fallopian tube on the side where no egg has been made will have a wasted journey. Others negotiate the tortuous part of the tube in the uterine wall and then arrive in the narrow part of the Fallopian tube.

Generally, the passage of fluid down the Fallopian tube is from the outer end to the inner, and from there to the uterus. However, at the time of ovulation the current of fluid is greatly reduced, so aiding the sperm's journey. The lining of the tube makes moisture, and the sperm actually travel up in the clefts of this greatly convoluted tube. The active sperm work their way up the far end of the Fallopian tube where the egg is waiting. By this time, no more than 100 of the original 200,000,000 sperm have reached the place where fertilization may occur. They then swarm around the egg.

Fertilization

Very soon one sperm penetrates the outer layer of the egg mass and its head is engulfed in the substance of the egg. The neck and tail are discarded and almost immediately, a biochemical barrier is erected around the whole substance of the egg to prevent any other sperm from penetrating. The nucleus of the sperm and that of the egg fuse, making a new cell which contains the genetic material of the mother's egg (1 out of 500,000) and of the father's sperm (1 out of 200,000,000).

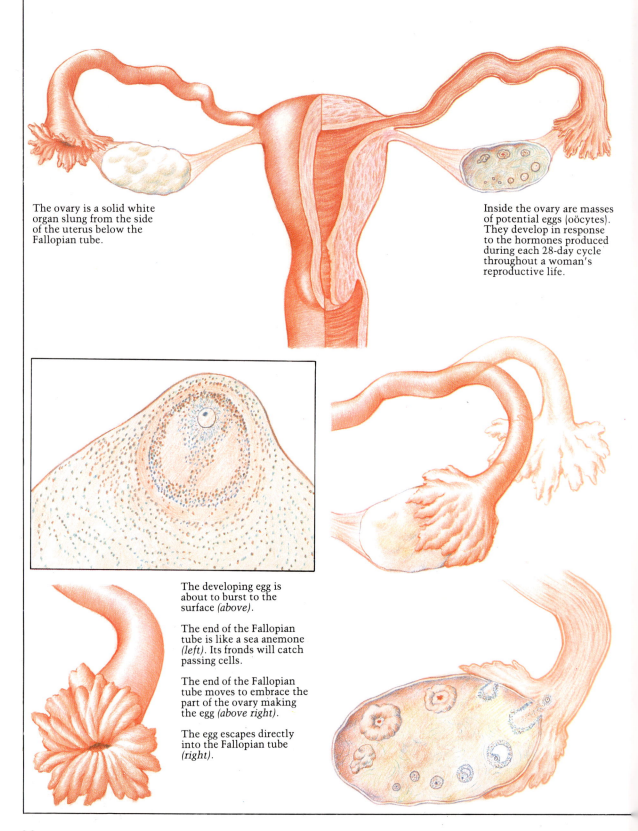

The ovary is a solid white organ slung from the side of the uterus below the Fallopian tube.

Inside the ovary are masses of potential eggs (oöcytes). They develop in response to the hormones produced during each 28-day cycle throughout a woman's reproductive life.

The developing egg is about to burst to the surface *(above)*.

The end of the Fallopian tube is like a sea anemone *(left)*. Its fronds will catch passing cells.

The end of the Fallopian tube moves to embrace the part of the ovary making the egg *(above right)*.

The egg escapes directly into the Fallopian tube *(right)*.

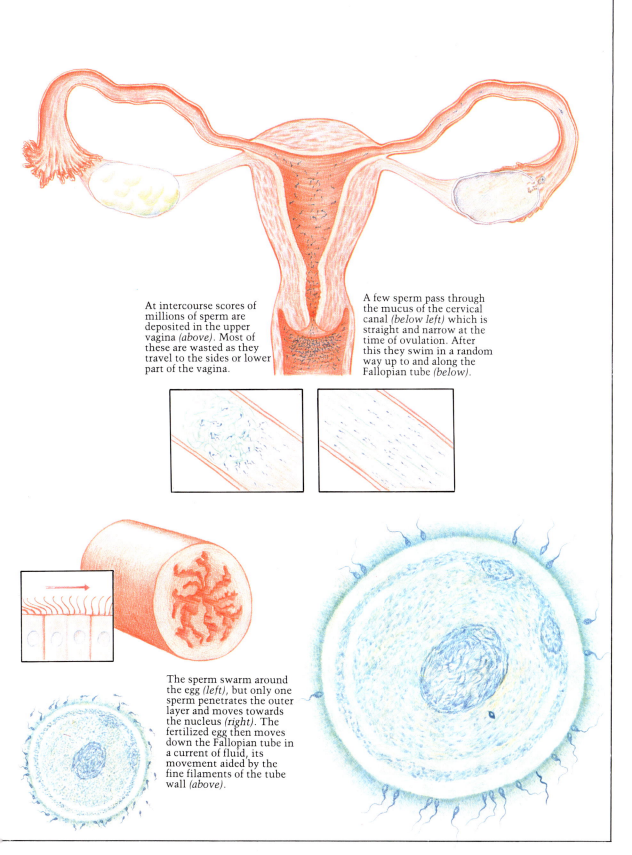

At intercourse scores of millions of sperm are deposited in the upper vagina *(above)*. Most of these are wasted as they travel to the sides or lower part of the vagina.

A few sperm pass through the mucus of the cervical canal *(below left)* which is straight and narrow at the time of ovulation. After this they swim in a random way up to and along the Fallopian tube *(below)*.

The sperm swarm around the egg *(left)*, but only one sperm penetrates the outer layer and moves towards the nucleus *(right)*. The fertilized egg then moves down the Fallopian tube in a current of fluid, its movement aided by the fine filaments of the tube wall *(above)*.

SEX OF YOUR BABY
This is determined by the sperm, about half of which are androgenic (making a male baby) and the other half gynogenic (making a female).

The androgenic sperm fare better in an acid environment than the gynogenic sperm. So, if you want a boy, you could use a mild acid gel or a vinegar douche in the vagina before intercourse. Similarly, a slightly alkaline environment favours gynogenic sperm; if you want a girl, you could try a bicarbonate of soda douche.

THE JOURNEY TO THE UTERUS

Two events then take place at the same time. The egg starts to roll slowly inside the tube and the vibrating hairs (cilia) on the tube's inner surface start to brush the fertilized egg down towards the uterus. As it progresses down the wider, outer part of the Fallopian tube, the single cell divides into two cells, the nucleus of each containing a complete reproduction of the total genetic material from the fused sperm and egg nuclei. This egg, now in its two-cell stage moves down the Fallopian tube propelled by the current fanned by the vibrating cilia and by muscular action at the outside of the tube massaging in a direction towards the uterus.

The egg then divides successively into four, eight and sixteen cells. After this, the cells go on dividing individually and there is no more mathematical precision. The rapidly growing bundle of cells soon resembles a mulberry and is called a morula, the name derived from the Latin word for this fruit. The morula passes from the Fallopian tube into the cavity of the uterus so that the egg is on the surface of the lining of the uterus by about Day 24 or 25 of the cycle in which fertilization occurred.

Single cell just after fertilization

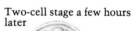

Two-cell stage a few hours later

Multiple-cell stage several days later

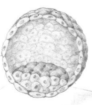

Cell group is divided into a cavity and a lower cell mass to become the baby

After fertilization, the nucleus of the sperm and the ovum fuse and the chromatin material from each of the nuclei join to make a new individual. This cell then passes down the Fallopian tube, dividing as it does into two, four, eight and more cells.

On entering the cavity of the uterus, the cell mass is too big to allow the innermost cells to exchange oxygen and carbon dioxide. In consequence, a cleft appears which soon becomes a cavity.

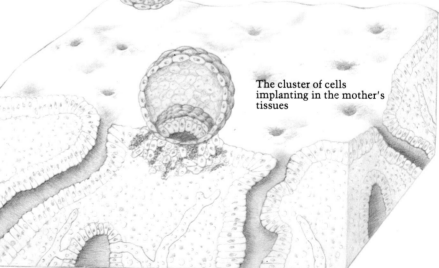

The cluster of cells implanting in the mother's tissues

Digestive hormones are then secreted from the morula so that the lining of the uterus gives way and the developing egg can snuggle down into the rich tissue. Since it is now about Day 25 or 26 of the cycle, the uterine lining is at its thickest and is ready to be implanted with the developed egg. Hormone signals from this egg to the ovary and the woman's pituitary gland prevent the usual menstrual cycle occurring and so generally no bleeding follows implantation.

Implantation

EMBRYONIC DEVELOPMENT

Development now continues quickly and the tissues of the embryo are laid down in an orderly fashion. The growth process is very rapid; a complex blueprint is made of the future embryo and soon the cells lose their contact with the outside world.

All the oxygen necessary for life and growth is obtained by diffusion on the surface of the cell bundle. Any waste products pass directly outwards from the cells through the same surface. Once the morula gets above a critical size, all the cells are no longer on the surface and they become a packed mass; a hollow sphere is formed and the fluid inside acts as a nutrient in the same way as that on the outside. A cleft appears in the middle of the mass so that all cells retain access to the surface, from which they can be nourished and get rid of their waste products. One part of the sphere thickens and develops into two layers and from this disc all tissues of the future baby develop.

Meanwhile, the whole mass of cells is buried in the uterine lining so that it is completely surrounded by the mother's tissues. For the next 38 weeks she provides the oxygen and nutrients required by the growing embryo, through the blood which surrounds it. At first, this interchange of nutrients and waste products between the embryo and the mother takes place all over the surface of the developing sac. To increase the surface area, the outside lining is thrown up into folds called villi which may act, in some instances, to anchor the growing embryo sac more firmly into the mother's tissues.

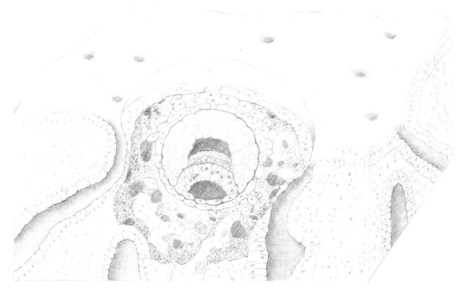

About eight or nine days after fertilization, the fetilized ovum settles on the surface of the uterus. Some of the cells on the surface of the fertilized ovum start eroding into the mother's tissues and the egg slowly settles into the mother's uterine lining. Soon blood vessels of the mother's uterus are opened and the mother's blood is allowed to circulate around the growing ovum. This is the source of nutrition for the embryo.

The placenta and umbilical cord

With increasing size, the sac containing the growing embryo bulges into the cavity of the mother's uterus whilst a smaller area covered by villi is in contact with the mother's blood. This area condenses down to a disc eventually covering about a quarter of the surface area of the sac and the disc becomes the placenta. All the communication between the growing fetus and the mother is concentrated through this. The placenta is the exchange station and the fetus's life depends upon it. Any alteration in exchange can affect the fetus, and a separation of the placenta from its bed on the uterine walls has serious results which may lead to a miscarriage.

Joining the placenta to the embryo is a leash of blood vessels. Blood is pumped from the fetus along both arteries to the placenta where it is re-oxygenated and the waste products are removed. It then returns along a vein back to the fetal circulation. These blood vessels are loosely bound together in the umbilical cord with a jelly that keeps them in position. The umbilical cord usually starts in the middle of the placenta and snakes its way through the fluid of the sac to the baby. It is quite slack and fairly long to allow the baby freedom of movement. At birth, the cord is usually about 80 cm in length but the range of variation is great and lengths from 10 to 150 cm have been measured in perfectly normal babies.

After a baby is born, the blood vessels in the umbilical cord go into spasm and shut tightly to minimize any loss of blood. In most other mammals, the cord is bitten through after delivery but in the human, the doctor or midwife clamps the umbilical cord to prevent any blood loss and cuts it. There are no

  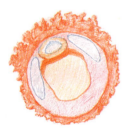 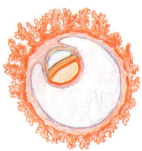

Once the sac containing the growing embryo has settled into the mother's uterine lining, the placenta begins to develop. It develops in accordance with the requirements of the fetus. All the substances the embryo receives from the mother and all its waste matter must pass through the 'placental barrier', so the fetus's life depends on it.

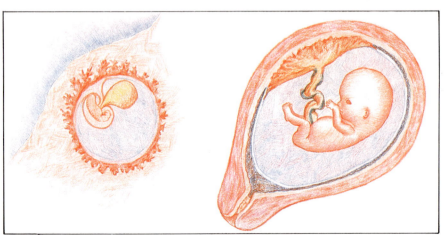

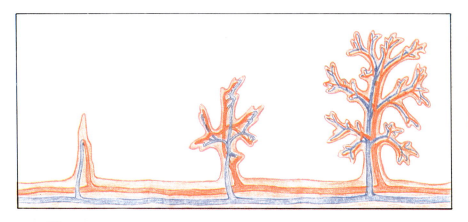

The blood vessels from the growing fetus develop in finger like processes in the placenta. This allows a greater surface area to be in contact with the mother's blood at the placental bed. Increased oxygen and food exchange is helped by the multiple branching of the placenta.

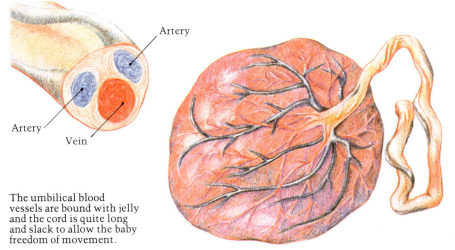

Artery

Artery

Vein

The umbilical blood vessels are bound with jelly and the cord is quite long and slack to allow the baby freedom of movement.

The embryo is joined to the placenta by a leash of blood vessels forming the umbilical cord. Blood is carried from the fetus along one of two arteries to the placenta where it is reoxygenated and waste products are removed. It then returns to the fetal circulation via the umbilical vein.

nerves in the cord and so no pain is felt by the baby or the mother when the bond that has held them together for 38 weeks is severed.

Amniotic fluid

The fetus develops in a fluid-filled sac, free from all attachments except the umbilical cord. His weight is supported by the fluid; he receives his oxygen from the placenta—not by breathing. He lives a relatively weightless existence, protected by the fluid from mechanical shocks and alterations of the mother's position; he is also cushioned from temperature changes and noise in this fluid environment.

The fluid is made mostly by the fetus himself, passing from his body across the very thin skin of the early embryo. Later it is made by the fetal kidneys while a third source is the lining membrane of the amniotic sac. The fluid constantly changes; it is disposed of by absorption across the same membranes around the sac and by the fetus swallowing. Thus he lives in a swimming pool of his own creation, the balance of which he determines. To be delivered, the baby obviously must leave his private swimming pool and the amniotic membrane over the neck of the dilating womb breaks, allowing some of the fluid to drain away. It is a clear, warm, slightly pungent fluid and no longer has a function in protecting the baby who is soon to be born.

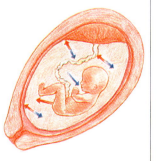

The amniotic fluid allows the fetus to float, protecting it from mechanical shocks and changes in temperature and sound.

DEVELOPMENT OF ORGANS

The implanted embryonic sac forms a disc of tissue in which the cells soon specialize into individual organs.

The brain and nervous system

About 15 days after conception, a rod of cells, which are on the surface of the disc and run along its length, start to thicken and then sink below the surface in a trough. The edges of this trough come together and seal off so that a tube is formed under the skin. This will be the baby's spinal cord. The sealing-up process starts in the lower back region moving upwards towards the head and downwards towards the tail end.

At the top end of this new tube, the nervous tissue expands both in width and length. Growth is limited by the size of the embryo and so the head end of the tube is bent forward and kinks, becomes convoluted and forms the complex pattern which becomes the brain. Two distinct bumps of tissue grow sideways from the front end of the central nervous tube and from them the very specialized upper brain, or cortex, is formed. This is where the higher thinking takes place and this area is connected to the rest of the nervous system by a series of complex cell pathways. The surface area of the brain becomes greatly increased inside the confines of the skull, so numerous folds are produced.

The brain communicates with all parts of the body, and the embryonic spinal cord sends out nerve processes, projections which grow into each limb and other organs. These strands of nervous tissue carry sensation from the organ to the nervous system, and different fibres in the same bundle carry electrical impulses out to the limbs and organs to make them work. All

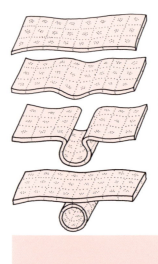

A groove of skin sinks in from the back of the embryo; soon it is sealed over, making a hollow tube This is the beginning of the spinal cord and central nervous system. At the head end, the tube is much more distended and enlarged making a larger mass of nervous tissue — the brain.

The hollow tube could go on expanding but this would be extravagant on space. Instead, the surface convolutes to allow for a lot of nervous tissue to occupy a small space inside the skull.

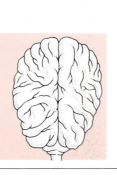

sensation comes into the nervous system and the instigation of all voluntary activity in the muscles and organs of the body proceeds from it. As each limb and organ develops, it carries these nervous processes with them; each part of the body needs nerves to be able to coordinate its activities with the other parts. By about 55 days of intrauterine life, the central nervous system and the nerves flooding to the other parts of the body have been formed.

The eyes

Each eye is formed by the expansion of a hollow nerve process which, as it approaches the skin of the face, becomes pushed in to form a cup. The skin over the cup then sinks to form the lens.

The ears

A similar pair of dips evolves to form the ear on each side of the head; a tube of skin from the throat grows out to meet a pocket of skin from the side of the head. These make the middle and outer ears. The inner ear, which provides balance and hearing, comes from an outgrowth of the nervous tissue of the brain which extends sideways to meet the two skin pouches. The outer flap of the ear which is seen prominently on the side of the head is made from several skin projections which fuse together.

The arms and legs

The elongated tube of the embryo develops limb buds just behind the head and halfway along the body by about the 30th day of life. These are tubes of skin filled with unspecialized tissue in which the bones and muscles of each limb are formed. Joints appear at the future ankles, knees, hips, wrists, elbows and shoulders, and around them ligaments condense to strengthen them. At first

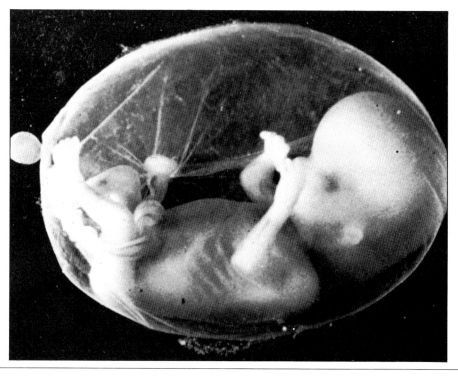

Limbs develop very early but are quite puny at first. The arm is more advanced than the leg in development but since they are not needed in the uterus, or in the early days of life, their full development is slow.

Joints in the limbs appear first of all as gaps between the bones (*right*).

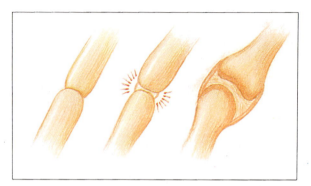

The digestive system develops from a simple tube which grows very rapidly. Since it is fixed at each end, many convolutions occur to accommodate the growth (*below*).

The hands and feet develop as paddles at the end of the limbs, (*right*) and separate into digits later.

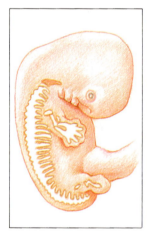

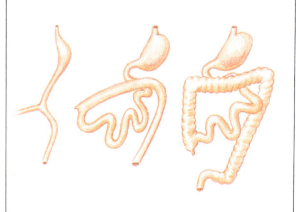

joints are simply gaps between the bones to allow a little bending to occur, but soon a more complicated arrangement is formed, and this is different for each joint. For example, the shoulder joint is a ball and socket, the socket part growing to embrace the ball to prevent dislocation. The bearing surfaces of each joint are covered with smooth cartilage to allow easy movement during the rest of life.

At the end of each limb, the tissues flatten out into a fan in which the small bones of the hand or foot differentiate. At first the fingers are joined together but soon they separate leaving only a small web of skin between them. The tips of the fingers and toes contain cells which have much thicker skin and which sink in, making the horny layer of the nails. At first this is covered by other skin but, before the baby is born, the nail has grown out to the end of each digit. In about 10 days, the limbs are formed with separate fingers and toes. Usually, arm development precedes that of the leg. Movements of the limbs start at about this time but cannot usually be detected by the mother until much later (16 to 20 weeks of pregnancy).

The digestive system

The digestive system develops from a simple tube from the mouth down to the anus. Since the tube grows more rapidly than the body around it, it can only find space by twisting and becoming convoluted. The tube is suspended from the back of the embryo's body and loops occur in it. Some parts of the tube increase in size to form the stomach and the large intestine.

The face

At the top end of the embryo the face is formed. The developing gut tube comes into contact with the area of skin at the head end. Just below the nose, a pit of skin sinks in to join the two and form the mouth cavity. The lips develop from bulges of skin that grow together; over the upper and lower rims of this cavity, tissue hardens to form first cartilage and then the bones of the jaws. Small pits of skin sink into this; later they form teeth that are really hard pegs of bone covered with enamel. From the floor of the mouth, a bridge of muscle expands upward to form the tongue, on which taste buds develop.

From either side of the space, a platform grows to form the floor of the nose and the roof of the mouth. The nose is made by fusion of the side buds of skin with the process that comes down from even further up on the head. The nostrils are formed and the upper lip becomes complete. The eyes start very far down and out on the face. As growth of the nose and upper lip proceeds rapidly the eyes achieve a higher position on the head and come closer together.

At the other end of the body the gut tube similarly joins a pit of tail skin to form the anus. Rings of muscle develop around this to become a sphincter controlling mechanism.

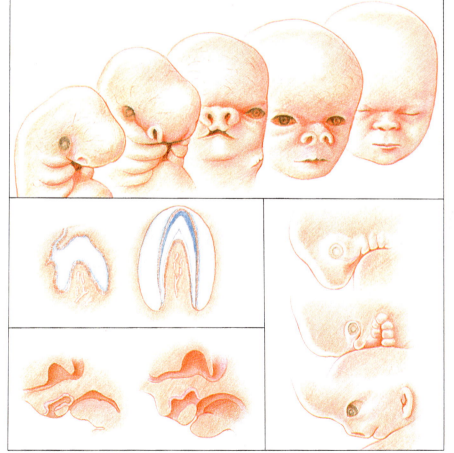

The face is formed from a series of stalks of skin coming from above and from the sides. The nose makes the central pillar downwards, the upper lip is formed from two ingrowths which fuse at the bottom of the nose.

The teeth sink into the gums as hard pegs of modified skin (enamel) which cover the inner sensitive area (dentine). The mouth joins the gut tube; the ears form low down on the sides of the head and migrate upwards.

The heart and blood vessels

Once the organism becomes so complex that the cells are no longer in contact with the surface, a system is developed to provide the cells with oxygen and nutrients and to get rid of the waste products. Internal circulation of the fluid is needed to link every cell with the body's oxygen and food supplies. This is the function of the blood stream; small vessels carry the blood to all parts of the body, returning it centrally. In the blood are red cells which carry the oxygen, while the basic foodstuffs are dissolved in the plasma for extraction by the individual cells.

About two weeks after conception, groups of blood-forming cells gather in islands in all parts of the body and these join together to form channels, making the arteries and veins. The central arteries run the length of the body just in front of the newly forming nervous system. In the chest area the tubes coalesce into a thick-walled organ which becomes the heart. Rapid growth of this tube, which is held firmly at each end, forms a sac (sacculation) which bends so that the kinks develop into valvular folds. This allows the blood to flow in one way only. A partition grows down the middle of the organ, dividing the heart into two sides, and the pumping action of the thickened muscle starts by about 22 days of life inside the uterus.

The heart is developed from a pair of blood vessels which fuse together and then grow in width and length. They are fixed at both ends and kink to form the heart as shown.

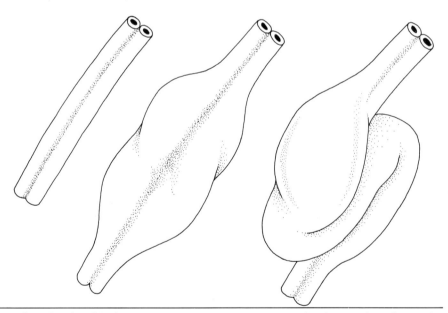

Respiration system

Before birth, the fetus receives oxygen, not via the lungs, but from the mother's own blood passed through the placenta. Lungs develop from pouches which have split off the gut tube and they make their own separate tubal system in front of the gut. They grow rapidly and convolute to form the spongy substance of the lung although they are not yet required and are unexpanded. The windpipe and the larger tubes are filled with lung liquid which is squeezed out of the lungs before breathing starts. In fact, the embryo does make some chest wall movements in the last weeks of pregnancy. These movements can be seen on an ultrasound machine and it is normal to expect such activity, for the fetus must practise breathing movements to be ready for the moment of birth when they will be essential to maintain life.

GROWTH OF THE FETUS

After the first eight or nine weeks of intrauterine life, the embryo is complete and the healthy fetus has all its essential organs. From now on time will be occupied with their growth and refinement. The rate of growth is very rapid, particularly in the middle months of pregnancy. At no other time in the rest of life will normal tissues grow as fast as this. If such a speed were to continue in later life, by the age of 21 the child would be as tall as Nelson's Column and would weigh several tons. Different parts of the body grow at different rates; the head end receives the most oxygenated blood so that the brain can grow quickly. This makes the developing embryo look big-headed in relation to the rest of its body. The limbs of the fetus look comparatively puny in relation to the body for they are little used. Once the baby starts to use them, months after birth, the limbs grow stronger and longer.

At conception, the fertilized egg weighs a few thousandths of a gram. When the child is born, he or she will weigh some three thousand grams (3 kg). This huge change in weight is made by the proliferation and growth of billions of cells. These must be laid down in an orderly fashion to produce a human being.

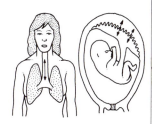

Adults exchange oxygen and carbon dioxide at the lungs (*above left*). The fetus has to do it at the placenta (*above right*) where, in addition, he exchanges all his foodstuffs.

The growth of the fetus is greater in the last weeks of pregnancy. The amount of fluid and the weight of the placenta also increases.

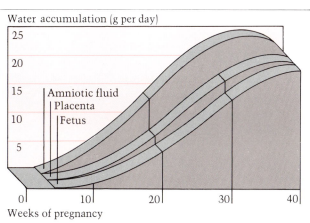

In absolute weight terms the fetus increases enormously compared to the placenta.

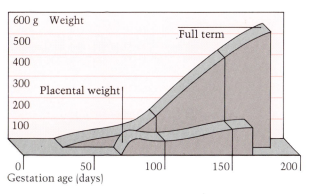

Some couples feel cheated if pregnancy does not come after two or three months of trying. But you must remember that only one egg a month is made and this lives for only 36 to 48 hours. The sperm which your partner makes lives for about 24 hours after ejaculation. So, unless the egg and sperm have been brought together in this very tight time zone in the middle of the cycle, you will not become pregnant during that month. Among normal couples using no contraception, about 80 per cent of the women will become pregnant after one year's unguarded intercourse and 90 per cent will be pregnant by the end of two years. If pregnancy is not achieved by this time you should consult your doctor.

If you decide that you need to seek formal help with conception your family doctor may do some tests to check your fertility and will probably refer you on to a specialist clinic for others. There are basically four areas that need to be assessed.

Ovulation

Doctors will want to know if you are making eggs. This can be checked by simple tests which examine aspects of your body's working to see if the hormone, progesterone, is released in the second half of the cycle. Of these tests, probably the simplest is the basal temperature chart. For this test you take your temperature first thing in the morning before rising from bed. If you record this each day you will see that your temperature is a little higher in the second half of the menstrual cycle than in the first half. This is most difficult to spot in prospect and you may need two or three months of charts before you get the hang of it.

Other ways of checking progesterone levels are to do a blood test in the latter part of the menstrual cycle or to check the cells from the wall of the vagina for the effect of the hormone changes on them. A curettage (D and C) may be carried out so that hormone changes reflected in the lining of the uterus can be examined. If ovulation is found to be deficient, your doctor can prescribe treatment to stimulate it. The treatment offered will be related to your particular deficiency, so do not think that the treatment given to your next-door neighbour would necessarily be helpful to you.

To see if you are ovulating you will need to fill in a basal temperature chart — two examples are shown here.

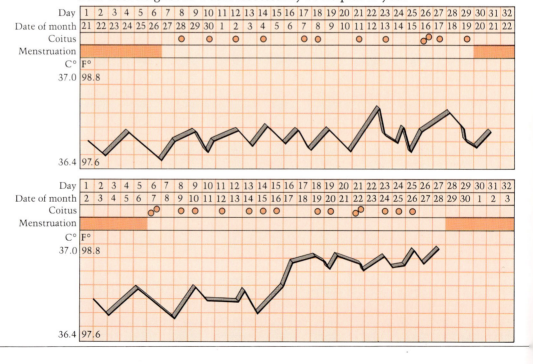

Making sperm

If you are concerned about fertility, you will have to consider not only your own ovulation, but also your partner's sperm-making capacity. It takes two to make a baby. The sperm check is quite simple: a masturbation specimen of semen, produced at home, is examined in the laboratory; the quantity, activity and shape of some of the sperm will be checked just to make sure that they are normal. While most men produce perfectly normal sperm, about a third of all couples attending infertility clinics (and for whom a diagnosis can be obtained) have a male feature of infertility. Often any reduction in sperm numbers or mobility can be improved by special hormone treatments.

Blockage of the tubes

The sperm and egg have to travel along the narrow Fallopian tubes in order to meet. The tubes are very easily blocked, particularly by infection, so the doctors will want to check that they are open. This can be done by bubbling some gas along them (insufflation) or more commonly by X-ray to outline them (hysterosalpingogram). In many centres the tubes can be seen with a special instrument—a laparoscope. The use of this requires a general anaesthetic and usually a night in hospital but it allows the infertility doctors to perform an excellent examination of the Fallopian tubes and the rest of the pelvis. Blockage of the Fallopian tubes may be correctable by an operation but results are not good. Talk carefully to your clinic doctors about this.

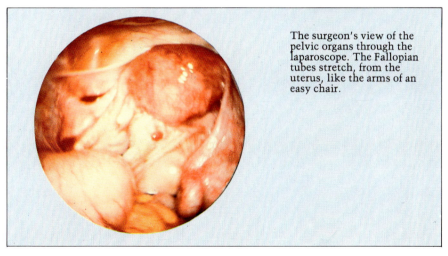

The surgeon's view of the pelvic organs through the laparoscope. The Fallopian tubes stretch, from the uterus, like the arms of an easy chair.

Interaction of male and female

More recently it has been realized that the woman may react against the male sperm and, indeed, that the man himself can make antibodies against his own sperm. Such paradoxes are not unknown in nature; a regular part of the fertility clinic's checks should be to see that there is no interaction between the two sets of tissues. Treatment is difficult and time-consuming but good results can be achieved.

These tests may seem complicated and, of course, they do intrude upon your privacy. However, you will no doubt readily understand that the doctors need information before they can be expected to diagnose or offer treatments. Accept the intrusions as best you can and take comfort from the fact that approximately 60 per cent of couples who attend an infertility clinic eventually produce healthy babies.

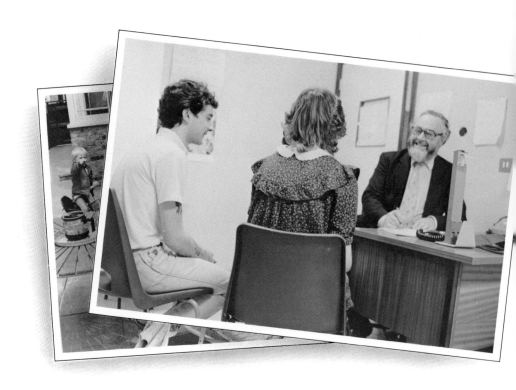

THE FIRST THREE MONTHS

Some of the first weeks of pregnancy will pass before you are actually certain that you are pregnant. However, if you have had a baby before you will probably know that you are pregnant in advance of a formal diagnosis. For most women there is a feeling of well-being and a sense of uplift; you will walk tall and feel very special. The first thing to do is to have your doctor confirm your pregnancy and then you can begin your formal antenatal care. This is the best way to safeguard the health of you and your baby.

DIAGNOSING PREGNANCY

Symptoms you notice

Most women are aware of the absence of menstruation; the date of the last normal period that occurred should be noted for this is useful later on. Some women, however, do not menstruate regularly every 28 days and so might be in some doubt as to whether the absence of a period is part of their normal pattern or not.

Very soon other changes will be noticed; the breasts become heavier and tender, often with a tingling sensation of the nipple area. As pregnancy proceeds, the breasts become larger and the nipple becomes darker. Little nodules appear in the nipple area and, later still, it is possible to press out some secretion from the breast which is the precursor to the milk.

Many women notice nausea in pregnancy by about the fifth or sixth week after the last normal menstrual period, that is two or three weeks after the first missed period. While this is commonly called morning sickness, it can occur at any time of day. The symptom passes by about the 12th to 14th week of pregnancy. It varies in severity but most women are not generally made very ill by this although it is a terrible nuisance (see pages 44 to 45).

Some find that they pass urine more frequently but there is usually no stinging or burning associated with this. It is a normal change following the hormone alterations to the body. The bladder becomes more sensitive and so responds more readily to a lesser volume of stored urine.

A woman who has had a child before will often notice she is pregnant very early after fertilization, for there is a general feeling which is hard to describe. Some consider it to be a feeling of well-being and are elated. Undoubtedly, the hormone changes of pregnancy occur very early and an experienced woman can spot this long before any of the more precise symptoms occur. An experienced doctor will pay attention to this vague sensation.

Signs the doctor notices

A doctor usually cannot distinguish pregnancy by examination until several weeks have gone by. The growing baby is tucked deep inside the uterus, which is itself in the bony pelvis. Most doctors do not make an examination until about 8 to 10 weeks, by which time the woman herself usually knows what is going on. After 12 weeks the uterus grows out of the bony pelvis and can be felt through the abdominal wall. The fetal heart beat cannot be

WHAT TO DO
When you think you are pregnant, make an appointment to see your GP at the next convenient surgery. Your doctor will probably want to do a pregnancy test, so take an early morning sample of urine with you. Once pregnancy has been confirmed your doctor will direct you towards systematic antenatal care; this will depend upon the facilities available in your area but probably you will be making an appointment for a booking visit at the hospital where you will deliver.

Early in your pregnancy you may notice a heaviness and a tingling sensation in your breasts.

detected with certainty by the ear until approximately 20 to 24 weeks have passed. However, the pulsations of the heart can be spotted with an ultrasound machine as early as 8 to 10 weeks of pregnancy.

Pregnancy tests

A simple laboratory test can be performed to confirm pregnancy. The test measures the level of the hormone—human chorionic gonadotrophin—in the body fluid, the most easily available of these being urine. The early morning specimen of urine is most concentrated and so this should be taken to your doctor or chemist for testing. There are also many good do-it-yourself tests which you can buy from the chemist. However, they are quite expensive and the instructions for carrying out the test are very detailed and must be followed exactly if an accurate result is to be had.

Provided there is an adequate concentration of hormone in the urine, pregnancy can be detected as early as 10 days after the missed period, that is about 22 days after conception or 38 days after the first day of the last normal menstrual period. If the test is negative it might mean there has not yet been enough time to get a high enough concentration of hormone and it should be repeated a few days later. By seven weeks after the first day of the last normal menstrual period the test is 99 per cent accurate.

THE TIMING OF PREGNANCY

Pregnancy lasts from the fertilization of the egg to delivery of the child. On average this is 38 weeks but it is quite normal for it to be a week or two either side of the precise day. About 90 per cent of women deliver within two weeks (either side) of this time.

Since intercourse may have taken place many times in a particular cycle the actual date on which a woman conceives is usually not known; the convention is to time the pregnancy from the first day of the last normal menstrual period, so that pregnancy is considered to be 40 weeks long, although it is obvious that for the first two weeks the woman is not pregnant.

Ovulation occurs 14 days before the next menstrual period, if a pregnancy does not follow. Intercourse must take place within 24 hours of ovulation for pregnancy to occur.

In the 30-day cycle shown, ovulation takes place approximately 16 days after the first day of the last period.

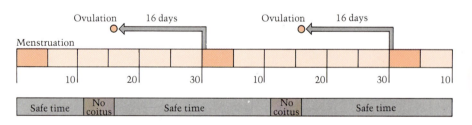

Pregnancy starts with fertilization of the egg and finishes with delivery of the baby. Fertilization occurs approximately 14 days after the first day of the last menstrual period.

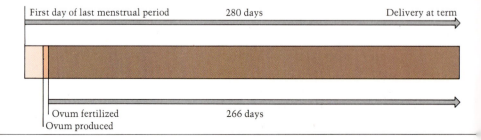

Do it yourself pregancy testing kits work in the same way as a laboratory test, by detecting the presence of pregnancy hormone in a woman's urine. This hormone starts to appear in the urine as soon as a woman becomes pregnant and can be dectected by a test as early as the first day after a missed period should have started.

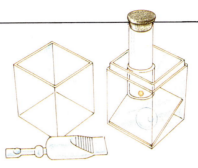

A typical kit consists of a test tube containing a pellet of the test reagent, resting in a holder with a mirror to read the result; a dropper tube containing liquid; and a box-shaped lid in which you pour a sample of the morning urine.

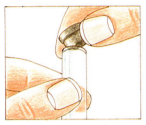

1 Take the test tube from its holder, remove the rubber stopper, then replace the tube in its holder.

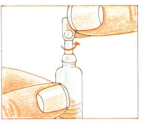

2 Take the dropper tube containing liquid from the holder and twist off the tip.

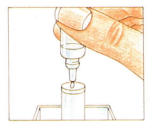

3 Squeeze all the liquid from the dropper tube into the test tube. Press the stopper back into the top of the test tube.

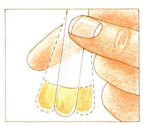

4 Shake the test tube until the contents are well mixed — at least 10 seconds. Put the test tube back into its holder.

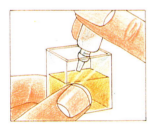

5 Squeeze the empty dropper tube to draw up some urine from the lid container.

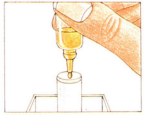

6 Add one drop only of the urine to the test tube, by gently squeezing the dropper tube.

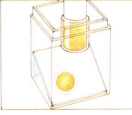

7 Put the stopper back in the test tube, shake the tube well and replace it in its holder.

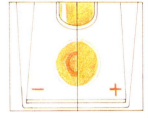

8 Two hours later — a dark brown ring means that you are not pregnant. An overall yellow-brown colour means that you are.

This applies to the majority of women who have a menstrual cycle of about 28 days. If, however, the cycle is irregular or prolonged this implies that egg-making is not in the middle of the cycle. Irrespective of the length of the cycle, the time from egg-making to the next menstrual period (or its absence in the case of pregnancy) remains a constant 14 days. Hence, for most, egg-making is 14 days before the next menstruation and 14 days after the last but if a woman has a 35-day cycle then the egg will not be made till Day 21. For such a woman, pregnancy will still be measured from the date of the last menstrual period but the expected delivery date will be later than that for a woman with a 28-day cycle.

The expected date of delivery can also be altered by other factors. If you have been taking the contraceptive pill until just before you become pregnant this may have altered your cycles so that the date will be less precise. Furthermore, if you should have some vaginal bleeding in early pregnancy,

DETERMINING YOUR DELIVERY DATE

January	1	2	3	4	5	6	7	8	8	10	11	12	13	14	15	16	17	18	19	20	21	22	23	24	25	26	27	28	29	30	31	January
October	8	9	10	11	12	13	14	15	16	17	18	19	20	21	22	23	24	25	26	27	28	29	30	31	1	2	3	4	5	6	7	November
February	1	2	3	4	5	6	7	8	9	10	11	12	13	14	15	16	17	18	19	20	21	22	23	24	25	26	27	28	29			February
November	8	9	10	11	12	13	14	15	16	17	18	19	20	21	22	23	24	25	26	27	28	29	30	1	2	3	4	5	6			December
March	1	2	3	4	5	6	7	8	9	10	11	12	13	14	15	16	17	18	19	20	21	22	23	24	25	26	27	28	29	30	31	March
December	6	7	8	9	10	11	12	13	14	15	16	17	18	19	20	21	22	23	24	25	26	27	28	29	30	31	1	2	3	4	5	January
April	1	2	3	4	5	6	7	8	9	10	11	12	13	14	15	16	17	18	19	20	21	22	23	24	25	26	27	28	29	30		April
January	6	7	8	9	10	11	12	13	14	15	16	17	18	19	20	21	22	23	24	25	26	27	28	29	30	31	1	2	3	4		February
May	1	2	3	4	5	6	7	8	9	10	11	12	13	14	15	16	17	18	19	20	21	22	23	24	25	26	27	28	29	30	31	May
February	5	6	7	8	9	10	11	12	13	14	15	16	17	18	19	20	21	22	23	24	25	26	27	28	1	2	3	4	5	6	7	March
June	1	2	3	4	5	6	7	8	9	10	11	12	13	14	15	16	17	18	19	20	21	22	23	24	25	26	27	28	29	30		June
March	8	9	10	11	12	13	14	15	16	17	18	19	20	21	22	23	24	25	26	27	28	29	30	31	1	2	3	4	5	6		April
July	1	2	3	4	5	6	7	8	9	10	11	12	13	14	15	16	17	18	19	20	21	22	23	24	25	26	27	28	29	30	31	July
April	7	8	9	10	11	12	13	14	15	16	17	18	19	20	21	22	23	24	25	26	27	28	29	30	1	2	3	4	5	6	7	May
August	1	2	3	4	5	6	7	8	9	10	11	12	13	14	15	16	17	18	19	20	21	22	23	24	25	26	27	28	29	30	31	August
May	8	9	10	11	12	13	14	15	16	17	18	19	20	21	22	23	24	25	26	27	28	29	30	31	1	2	3	4	5	6	7	June
September	1	2	3	4	5	6	7	8	9	10	11	12	13	14	15	16	17	18	19	20	21	22	23	24	25	26	27	28	29	30		September
June	8	9	10	11	12	13	14	15	16	17	18	19	20	21	22	23	24	25	26	27	28	29	30	1	2	3	4	5	6	7		July
October	1	2	3	4	5	6	7	8	9	10	11	12	13	14	15	16	17	18	19	20	21	22	23	24	25	26	27	28	29	30	31	October
July	8	9	10	11	12	13	14	15	16	17	18	19	20	21	22	23	24	25	26	27	28	29	30	31	1	2	3	4	5	6	7	August
November	1	2	3	4	5	6	7	8	9	10	11	12	13	14	15	16	17	18	19	20	21	22	23	24	25	26	27	28	29	30		November
August	8	9	10	11	12	13	14	15	16	17	18	19	20	21	22	23	24	25	26	27	28	29	30	31	1	2	3	4	5	6		September
December	1	2	3	4	5	6	7	8	9	10	11	12	13	14	15	16	17	18	19	20	21	22	23	24	25	26	27	28	29	30	31	December
September	7	8	9	10	11	12	13	14	15	16	17	18	19	20	21	22	23	24	25	26	27	28	29	30	1	2	3	4	5	6	7	October

To find out when your baby is due you need to know the first day of your last period. Find this date along one of the top (black) rows in the chart. The date you should deliver your baby is given immediately underneath in the brown numbers. So, for example, if the first day of your last period was 1 January, your expected delivery date is 8 October.

something that happens to about one in ten women, this may be mistaken for the last proper menstrual period and would alter the timing.

It is important to have a note of the first day of the last normal menstrual period so that these calculations can be made. If you are trying to conceive, you should get into the habit of keeping such dates in your diary.

GROWTH OF THE BABY

In Chapter 2 you can see in detail the growth of the individual organs and the whole fetus. The opposite page shows the actual size of the baby in the weeks of pregnancy with which we are dealing in this section.

You will see that these drawings show a very small baby, but at about 10 weeks he is complete with all his organs. The remainder of the gestation period is devoted to the growth and development of these organs.

CHANGES IN THE MOTHER

As well as pleasant changes you may also have some less happy ones. The most common of these is nausea. This may start as a simple aversion to certain foods or alcohol. It often occurs early in the day and so is known as

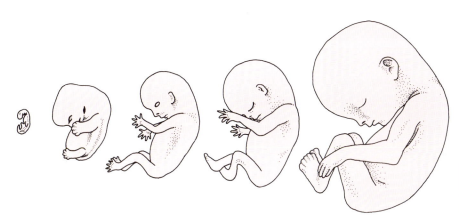

The fetus grows very rapidly in size and complexity in early pregnancy. These life-size drawings show the fetus from 3 to 12 weeks after fertilization.

morning sickness, but a large number of women suffer nausea at other times as well. The best cure is to ensure that the stomach is not completely empty before any nausea occurs. If you are suffering from morning sickness, you could ask your partner to bring you tea with a biscuit or piece of toast to take before you get up. This will at least help to relieve the symptoms. Similarly, during the day, large meals should be avoided but small meals should be taken frequently. Any thoughts of weight control should be put to one side at this stage and you should eat what you can in reasonable quantities in order to keep something in the stomach. If the vomiting is severe, you should consult your doctor.

Many women feel a great emotional upheaval at this stage and some find themselves unable to concentrate on their jobs. Even if you are really happy to be pregnant, it is quite usual to feel a temporary depression, to be moved to tears easily or even to be bad-tempered and irritable. A general lassitude is also very common. These feelings are easily explained by altered hormone levels and by the drain on your physical resources which the growing embryo is making at this time. Happily, this period is short-lived and a stage of contentment should follow..

A few women have unusual and exotic appetite desires, this is called *pica*. They seek out foods or combinations of foods which they do not normally eat. The fulfilment of these cravings used to be much more difficult, but now, with deep frozen foods at every large supermarket, it is difficult for a woman's *pica* to outrun the grocer's supplies.

A general feeling of emptiness in the stomach is more common and is sometimes difficult to control. Some women have an acute appetite increase which can only be satisfied by eating enormous quantities of bulky food such as bread or vast quantities of cakes or biscuits. This should be controlled as much as possible as there is no need to take in large amounts of carbohydrates at this stage. If a craving does exist, it would be better to try fruit or salads to fill the gap.

Some women also notice a slight watery mucous discharge from the vagina. This is quite normal, for the glands at the neck of the womb are making more mucous. If, however, this condition is also irritant, it implies that an infection in the vagina may have followed and this should be investigated.

WHY ARE YOU SICK IN EARLY PREGNANCY?

During pregnancy about two-thirds of women are sick, not always in the moring. This is probably due to a rise in the level of the hormone, chorionic gonadtrophin, produced by the growing embryo in large amounts. Its secretion regulates many functions in the body and ensures that the developing infant stays in the uterus in the first few weeks of pregnancy. Once fetal growth is established, by about 10 to 12 weeks, the concentrations of the hormone are reduced and the sickness commonly gets better.

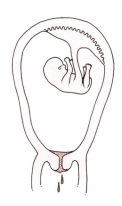

The cervix produces a lot of mucus during pregnancy.

WHY GO FOR ANTENATAL CARE?

During pregnancy, the normal woman consults her general practitioner, obstetrician and midwives even if she has no major problems. They are part of a preventative health service which tries to prevent problems ocurring or, at least, to arrest them early if they should arise. During antenatal care it is hoped that you will be able to get to know the team of people who will be looking after you. Antenatal care is important for the following reasons:

1 Any symptoms (eg pain or bleeding) which worry a woman during pregnancy can be treated at an early stage.

2 It provides a screening service to prevent problems; regular examinations would detect abnormal conditions early (eg toxaemia of pregnancy).

3 It provides the woman and her partner with the potential to learn more about pregnancy and childbirth.

When do you go?

Once you have consulted your family doctor and your pregnancy has been confirmed you will have to decide where you would like the delivery to be. Eighty per cent of women in the UK choose the local hospital, about 15 per cent a GP unit, which may be associated with that hospital, and the remainder select other places, such as private accommodation or the home. When you have decided, you will be referred for a booking visit at the antenatal clinic associated with the agreed place. Although you may attend the hospital for a booking visit, you may not have to go there for all antenatal visits and may share care between the hospital and your GP. This is the arrangement for about half the women who eventually deliver in hospital.

NATIONAL CHILDBIRTH TRUST

NCT classes allow for small groups of pregnant women and their partners to meet regularly for six weeks in an informal setting. The size of the group allows for trust and confidence to build up and for firm friendships to develop. You can feel free to raise any of the hopes or fears that concern you during your pregnancy, and you can learn from others' experiences.

One of the aims is to teach a method of relaxation which will allow you to remain in control during your labour (see pages 62 to 63 for relaxation exercises). These classes also give you the oportunity to learn more about the choices that are available to you, eg the drugs, the positions for delivery etc, so that you have all the information necessary to make an informed choice.

Just as important as the preparation for childbirth is the support system available once your baby is born. If you attend classes you will automatically be put in touch with one of the local post-natal supporters. She may be of some help to you in the early weeks and will be able to put you in touch with specialist help should you have particular problems.

What do you do at the booking clinic?

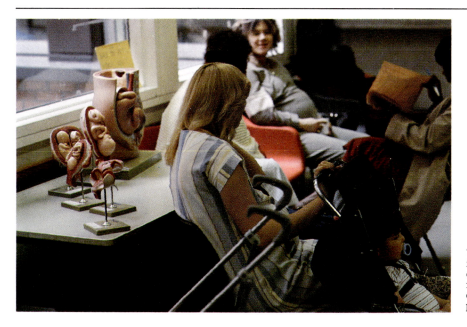

The booking clinic is the first, and most important, of the many visits you will make to the antenatal clinic during your pregnancy.

The principal event at the booking clinic is meeting the team who will be looking after you in pregnancy and labour. You will meet one of the senior midwives in the team, some of the junior midwives and probably one of the doctors. This is the longest hospital visit and probably the most important, but it can be tiresome waiting around if you are not prepared for it. Most booking clinics take up two to three hours; during this time you will go through all the details of your past health and present problems so that you can get on the right track for this pregnancy. Try to be patient on this first visit; take something good to read with you and arrive there being prepared to stay for several hours.

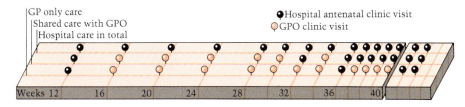

Antenatal care may be with your GP and his community midwife, shared with the hospital or at the hospital only.

Medical history

One of the midwives will talk to you about your medical history. You need not worry about talking freely to her; everything you say will be treated in strict confidence within the hospital and may be of great value to the medical team in the management of your pregnancy and the health of your future baby. It would be important for them to know, for example, if you had had any back or spinal problems; you might not immediately see the relevance of this information, but the medical team would realize that this could affect the passage of the baby through the pelvis during labour. Similarly, the midwife will ask about the family medical history. She will want to know if there is a history of diabetes or twins, for both have a recurrence rate in the family and both need to be detected early.

If you have had a previous pregnancy, the midwife will ask you about this. She will want to know about any problems in that pregnancy, the stage in pregnancy the baby was born, the events of delivery and the birthweight of the baby; how you were after the delivery and how the baby progressed. She will also need to ask questions about any pregnancy that did not proceed such as spontaneous or induced miscarriages. This may be a subject which is difficult for you to talk about but it is very important that the medical and midwifery staff have all the information available so that they can help both you and your unborn child through *this* pregnancy.

You will also be asked about the timing of the last menstrual period. Do not be concerned if, as well as asking about this date, she asks about the cycle of periods beforehand — as we have already, seen some women do not have 28-day cycles and others have a little bleeding after pregnancy starts. The midwife will discuss this aspect in detail, as it is an important matter to record in the notes while it is still fairly fresh in the memory.

General examination

You may wonder why you have to have a medical examination when you feel, after all, perfectly fit. The reason is simply to confirm that this really is so. Pregnancy and childbirth are physically demanding experiences and it is as well to be sure of your health from the outset. The doctor will check that there is no anaemia by looking at the thin skin of the lower eyelid and will then probably take your blood pressure. There is no one accepted level for blood pressure, but by recording your blood pressure now, the doctor can ensure that it is within an accepted range of normality. He then has a standard against which he can assess any fluctuation which might occur during your pregnancy.

The heart and lungs will also be examined. In the vast majority of women these are perfectly normal. However, the doctor will want to eliminate the

---

WHY IS ANAEMIA BAD?

Anaemia is a reduction in the amount of haemoglobin circulating in the blood; this is bad for the mother since it allows less oxygen to be carried to the tissues that need it. Even when we are sitting down our muscles are quietly working and using a little oxygen; we are constantly using oxygen for vital processes such as the beating of the heart and the digestion of food. When we get up and move around, we require even more oxygen, therefore, if you are anaemic, you will become tired more rapidly.

The fetus can suffer from the mother's anaemia for all his oxygen must be obtained through her; if she is anaemic he is likely to become chronically short of oxygen. Furthermore, anyone who is short of haemoglobin is likely to be short of other blood constituents.

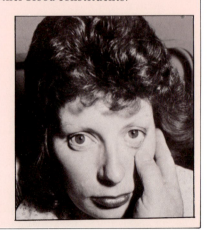

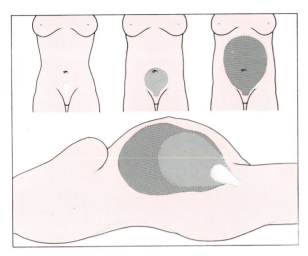

Growth of the uterus at 12, 25 and 36 weeks of pregnancy (*left*).

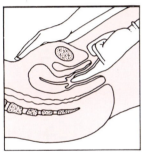

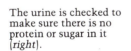

A vaginal assessment may be made to check that the uterus is enlarged and there are no abnormal masses (*left*).

The urine is checked to make sure there is no protein or sugar in it (*right*).

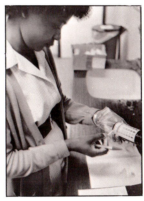

slight possibility of an unsuspected disease of these organs. Most doctors also check the spine to ensure that it is normal and that there are no points of weakness. Pregnancy can lead to spinal difficulties, as hormones produced in the fetus allow softening of the ligaments that support the spine; any pre-existing spinal problem will be exacerbated during pregnancy.

Your weight will also be checked. It would be ideal to know your pre-pregnancy weight; if you have a record of this, take it with you to the booking clinic to tell the doctors. Naturally, your weight will increase during pregnancy because of the growing baby and its support system, but there are reasonable limits within which you should try to stay.

The doctor will usually check the stomach to make sure that there are no undesirable lumps such as fibroids of the uterus. It is not usually possible to feel the growing uterus coming up out of the pelvis at this stage (normally about 12 weeks). The uterus is tucked away in the pelvis, the bony cage at the bottom of the stomach. To examine it the doctor inserts one or two fingers into the vagina and presses upward while his other hand presses downward on to the growing uterus. Your doctor will be able to detect this swelling and to determine how far pregnancy has progressed. No vaginal examination is pleasant, but the first one of pregnancy is very important for it enables the doctor to give a reasonable confirmation of the date on which the baby might be expected. Furthermore, it is important to check that there are no other lumps in the pelvis such as a small cyst in the ovaries or a fibroid in the uterus. The capacity of the bony pelvis is not normally checked.

Blood pressure is checked at every visit to the antenatal clinic. This is an important preventative measure to ensure that pre-eclampsia does not develop.

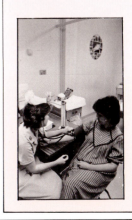

The tests done

SICKLE CELL ANAEMIA
This inherited condition is found almost exclusively in negroes. It is due to abnormal molecules of haemoglobin being present in the blood and can only be inherited if both parents have the sickle cell tendency. Haemoglobin carries oxygen to the tissues and when oxygen levels are reduced, the abnormal haemoglobin causes the red cells to be deformed into a sickle shape and these are then destroyed. This leads to a severe anaemia and to blood clots occuring in the small vessels of the body.

Human beings differ from other species in that their blood is divisible into groups which cannot be mixed. The main groups in the human are known by the A, B and O classifications. Of these the commonest is group O; about 47 per cent of us belong to this group. Group A is the next most common with 42 per cent. Groups B and AB are much rarer with 8 and 2 per cent respectively. It is important to know a woman's group in pregnancy, for she may need a blood transfusion urgently during labour.

The booking visit is the beginning of a series of tests which continue throughout pregnancy to ensure the good health of you and your baby. Both your blood and urine will be checked at regular intervals. Urine tests are best carried out on a sample passed first thing in the morning for this is the most concentrated. Two aspects are commonly checked:

1 The presence of glucose in the urine. This would imply an upset in the metabolism of the carbohydrate and that both mother and fetus were at risk. A positive result does not necessarily mean diabetes but the fetus should be subject to greater vigilance to spot any abnormal growth patterns. This is an easy test to carry out and much information can be deduced from it.

2 The presence of protein in the urine. In early pregnancy, this indicates an infection of the urinary tract. In later pregnancy this can be one of the warning signs of toxaemia, a progressive condition which affects both the mother and the baby (see pages 90 to 91). It is wise to make sure that there is no protein in the urine early in pregnancy so that, should it be found later, it will be known to be a result of the pregnancy and not a pre-existing condition.

A small sample of blood is taken at the booking visit. This hardly hurts at all and yields valuable results in the subsequent care of the mother and unborn child. It may seem a lot at the time, in fact, it is only 10 ml and the body replaces this within a few minutes. This small sample is sufficient for all the tests of early pregnancy. When the blood reaches the laboratory it is divided up and the different tests are carried out.

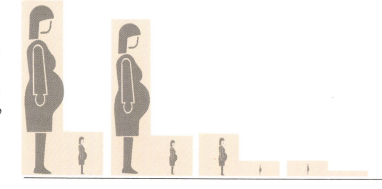

1 The haemoglobin level is checked. Haemoglobin is the red pigment which carries oxygen around the body in the blood and stops you becoming anaemic. If the level drops too low it may be dangerous to the mother and her unborn child. Should anaemia be detected in early pregnancy there is plenty of time to correct it with relatively simple treatments.

2 The blood group is checked. The correct grouping must be known in case a transfusion is needed following blood loss in later pregnancy. In addition, the rhesus grouping is tested; this is discussed fully on pages 75 to 77.

Many hospitals check the blood level of the chemical alpha fetoprotein. A high level can indicate spinal problems in the unborn baby. This is discussed fully on page 73.

Those who come from parts of the Mediterranean area or Africa sometimes have a weakness in the blood cells which leads to their collapse, so that the cells are no longer round and target-like, but look like half-moons or sickles. The incidence of sickling is higher in those whose ancestors originate from the Mediterranean basin; it is wise to know about this before pregnancy progresses too far so that extra antenatal care can be given and preparations can be made for the delivery. Only those in the group at risk will be tested for this.

German measles is a common infection in youth and, by the time of pregnancy, 85 per cent of women have had the condition. The level of antibodies is checked in early pregnancy to ensure the presence of a reasonable concentration. This then provides protection to both mother and unborn child during this pregnancy. If there are insufficient antibodies, immunization with German measles vaccine should be offered after this pregnancy, for future protection.

In many countries, a full chest X-ray is taken in early pregnancy to look for evidence of tuberculosis. This is so rare now in this country that most units do not offer a chest X-ray to any woman unless there is a family history of the condition.

What do you gain from the booking visit?

Firstly, and most importantly, you will meet the team in the hospital. They will, of course, be busy but if you have questions about pregnancy or childbirth to ask them they will be glad to talk to you. You will probably meet these people many times during the course of your pregnancy so you need not ask all the questions on this first visit. You may find it helpful to make out a list of questions *before* you go to this and subsequent clinics. It is all too easy to forget what you want to ask, once you are caught up in the bustling and unfamiliar atmosphere of the hospital.

At the booking clinic you will also be put in touch with the medical social workers. They will advise you about the benefits to which you are entitled. Every woman who is pregnant is entitled to some social security benefits. You should take these, for the taxes which you and your partner have paid over the years entitle you to them. If you feel you do not need the money, you could put it into a savings account for your child for the future.

Advice will be given about visiting the dentist. During pregnancy, any caries of the teeth proceeds very rapidly because they have a reduced resistance to infection. For this reason teeth deteriorate more rapidly at this time than at any other. Dental treatment is free during pregnancy and for one year afterwards; you should take advantage of this and get yourself into good shape.

Finally, at the booking clinic you will be given a fistful of leaflets concerning all sorts of events. You will be told about the local arrangements for maternity care, the social security benefits and the antenatal instruction classes. You will be given advice about your diet, activity and exercises (see also pages 13 to 16) and finally a bottle of iron tablets. The visit will have taken two hours or so and you will have met many people. You will probably be slightly bewildered by this time but these pages should help you to understand some of the reasons for the various activities. The medical team will be bustling about their jobs doing what to them is an everyday function, but everyone knows that to you it is a very special occasion.

See your dentist at least once during pregnancy; visits during pregnancy (and for a year afterwards) are free, and caries might get worse during this time.

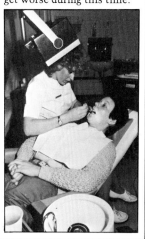

PROBLEMS THAT MAY ARISE

Bleeding in early pregnancy

Some pregnancies are destined not to continue. Usually this follows some maldevelopment of the growing embryo incompatible with life, and nature therefore decides to stop the pregnancy. This leads to a miscarriage with expulsion of the embryo, its membranes and the placenta from the uterus. While this is distressing for the woman who has looked forward to getting pregnant, in the long term perhaps it is for the best, for it means that she will not give birth to a malformed baby.

Threatened miscarriage

Sometimes, however, the uterus, even with a normal baby inside, just threatens to miscarry. There may be some bleeding from the vagina without any pains or cramps. In this event you should seek medical advice fairly soon. The doctor, in the home or in the hospital, gently examines to see if the neck of the womb is closed. If the cervix is not open then there is a good chance of the pregnancy continuing for it means that the embryo is not too badly affected and expulsion is by no means certain. Bed rest is the best treatment and

Occasionally, a very early miscarriage threatens. If the neck of the womb is closed, there is a chance that the pregnancy will continue (*right*). If the neck of the womb opens, the miscarriage is inevitable and the embryo will be lost (*far right*). If the fetus settles in the Fallopian tube (*bottom*), it may grow for a few weeks but no longer than this. Eventually, it will burst the tube and cause the problems of an ectopic pregnancy.

MISCARRIAGE

A miscarriage is a shock no matter how early in your pregnancy it happens; after the joy of conception you are suddenly left empty again. No words can take away the pain, but it will probably help you to cope with the loss if you can discuss your feelings with your partner, your doctor and your close friends. Your doctor will be able to advise and reassure you about your next pregnancy, and your friends, even if they feel that they don't know what to say to you, will allow you to unburden yourself.

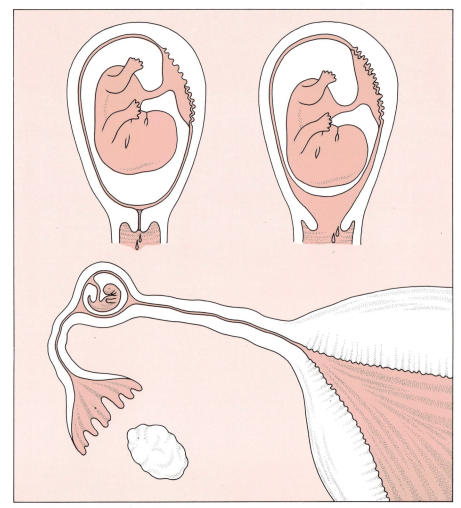

should last until at least 48 hours after the last fresh red bleeding. Treatment may be at home or, if the family doctor is concerned, in hospital for greater security. If bleeding happens repeatedly it should be accepted that this pregnancy is more at risk than others and it would be wise to give up some activities in the home or workplace in order to rest more than others would. This is an individual need and so should be judged individually for each woman, by the woman herself, by her own doctor and by an obstetrician.

Inevitable miscarriage

If the process of miscarriage has gone further and the embryo is certain to be expelled, the neck of the womb opens; the doctor can tell this at an internal examination. With the neck of the womb open, the contents have either been expelled or are about to be when he examines her. This is potentially a more dangerous situation for the woman than that of threatened miscarriage. She needs to be admitted to hospital straight away, for the amount of bleeding could be considerable; she should be under the care of a specialist gynaecologist who will be able to prevent more bleeding or to deal with it when it comes. This is an inevitable miscarriage and needs full hospital attention.

When the embryo is expelled the woman may not notice it for there is a lot of clot and blood around. Often the membranes or a part of the still-forming placenta are retained inside the uterus. If these were to remain, they would form the nidus for infection and allow even more bleeding; consequently, most hospital doctors would advise any woman who has an inevitable abortion, even if she has passed the embryo, to have a small operation to evacuate the remains of clot and membrane from the uterus. This is like a curettage or D and C and is called an Evacuation of Retained Products. It involves a light anaesthetic and takes about 10 minutes. It is important for the future reproductive state of the woman for the uterus to be emptied to allow the next pregnancy to start on a healthy organ.

Very occasionally, an infection follows either an inevitable or a complete abortion; this can lead to a woman being very ill and requiring antibiotics and intensive treatment in hospital. If this is done promptly then future fertility need not be impaired, but quick and full attention is imperative.

Ectopic pregnancy

The vast majority of pregnancies start inside the uterus when the fertilized egg moves down the Fallopian tube and enters that organ at about the seventh day after fertilization. However, a small number of eggs remain in the Fallopian tube where they are delayed. They then implant in the tube itself. The lining of the tube is not so thick as that of the uterus and cannot deal with the expanding egg nor the increased demands made upon the tissues for a greater supply of blood. In consequence, after a few weeks, the egg sac ruptures through the tube into the stomach cavity. This is accompanied by a severe pain and considerable loss of blood, so that the woman becomes very shocked and ill. This is a major catastrophe in a woman's life and an urgent operation will be needed to clamp off the bleeding area. Sadly, this often means the removal of the Fallopian tube from that side. However, a woman who has had an ectopic pregnancy and removal of the tube need not feel that the future is black. Her chances of another normal and intrauterine pregnancy are greater than 70 per cent and it is on this that she should pin her hopes.

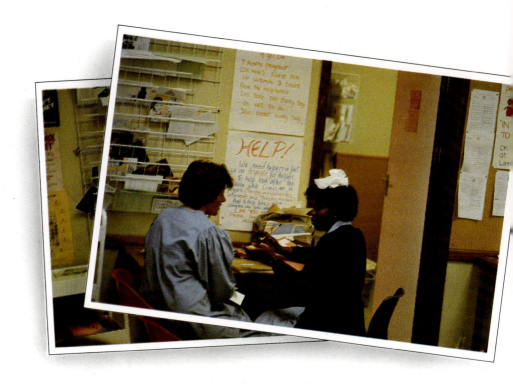

THE MIDDLE MONTHS

The middle third of pregnancy is the safest time for the mother and baby. The active development of the organs of the unborn baby has now finished and he is growing rapidly. The baby has a great influence on the mother's body long before his size causes the uterus to stretch so much that she can be aware of his presence. From very early in pregnancy the fetus is producing a series of chemical signals — hormones — which pass across the placenta into the mother's circulation. These cause adaptations in the function of many organ systems. These changes probably have evolved to minimize the stress of pregnancy imposed upon the woman's body; on the whole they are inter-locked smoothly with the efficient function of all the woman's body changes during pregnancy.

THE ADAPTATION OF THE WOMAN'S BODY

When the growing embryo is very small, he makes a hormone called chorionic gonadotrophin, a powerful chemical that reacts with many tissues of the body. One of the less pleasant side effects may be that of nausea in early pregnancy. Another more obviously beneficial one is that it helps the uterus to adapt to the growing sac of the embryo so that it does not contract prematurely and expel the enlarging clump of cells. Other fetal hormones are soon added. They are principally oestrogens, made by the growing tissues of the fetus, and progesterone — made at first by the remnant of cells left in the ovary from which the egg came (corpus luteum) and later by the placenta growing with the fetus. These and other hormone signals have profound effects on the mother's body. There is an increase in the load on the whole body of the pregnant woman. As well as the obvious increase in the uterus, all muscles get a little heavier, fat stores are increased, and the heart has to work harder to pump the blood to all parts of the body to provide the extra oxygen required. Furthermore, the fetus, and his wrap-around protective muscular uterus, demand a large share of the blood supply; the fetus for his growing body and the uterine muscles for the oxygen and nutrients they need.

Load on the heart

Most women gain between 10 to 15 kg during pregnancy. This leads to increased muscular activity and a greater blood supply. Because of this the output of the heart is increased greatly. The output of the heart can be measured by the amount of blood pumped at each beat of the heart, multiplied by the number of times it beats per minute (the pulse rate). In pregnancy, the heart rate is slightly raised, but most of the increase in cardiac output comes from the larger volume expelled at each stroke. The heart enlarges and its chambers get bigger. The muscle fibres of the heart strengthen and lengthen. In all, the heart pumps out each minute about 40 per cent more blood than it would before pregnancy, this rise occuring fairly early on, so that by about 16 weeks of pregnancy most of the increase in heart load has taken place. It is then maintained at the new level for the rest of pregnancy. In addition, during labour itself the cardiac output can increase by another 20 to 30 per cent with uterine contractions. The volume of blood occupying the blood vessels increases and the resistance of the small blood vessels all over the body slightly diminishes.

Blood is made up of both fluid (plasma) and cells, the most numerous of which are the red cells which bear the haemoglobin, the pigment which

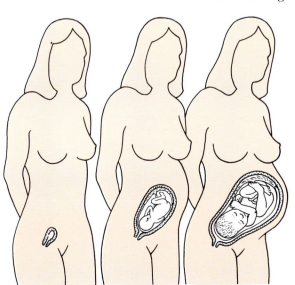

The growth of the uterus during pregnancy causes an alteration in the bulge of the stomach and the arching of the mother's back.

Cardiac output may increase by 40 per cent in the first 20 weeks of pregnancy. The uterine blood flow starts to increase sharply from the 20th week, to allow for the rapidly growing fetus. By the end of pregnancy, blood flow can be over 600 ml (more than a pint) a minute.

Uterine blood flow frequency

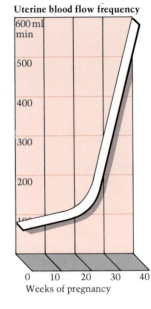

Weeks of pregnancy

Increased cardiac output

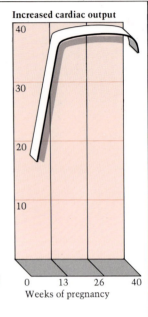

Weeks of pregnancy

CHRONIC SKIN DISEASE IN PREGNANCY

In the pregnancy age group, most skin diseases are not serious ones. However, if you had a chronic skin disease before pregnancy it could become a great irritation by flaring up in pregnancy. The two most common symptoms are itch and burning of the skin. In addition there may be blotchy discolouration of areas of the skin with raised scaling. Uncommonly there are weeping areas of skin in pregnancy.

During pregnancy a few skin diseases get a little better for the increased level of natural steroids made by the mother sometimes eases them. If they do not, you should consult your doctor who can provide you with more effective treatments that do not affect the unborn child.

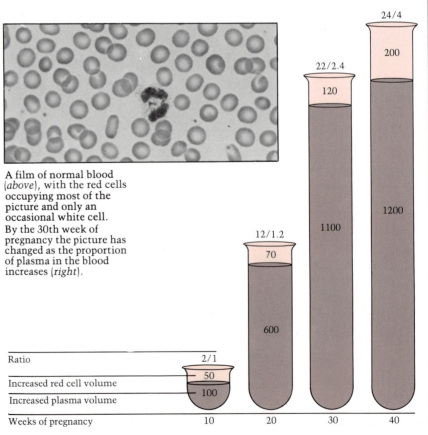

A film of normal blood (*above*), with the red cells occupying most of the picture and only an occasional white cell. By the 30th week of pregnancy the picture has changed as the proportion of plasma in the blood increases (*right*).

Ratio		2/1	12/1.2	22/2.4	24/4
Increased red cell volume		50	70	120	200
Increased plasma volume		100	600	1100	1200
Weeks of pregnancy		10	20	30	40

carries oxygen around the body. The increase in the fluid component of blood is slightly greater than that of cells; it is easier for the body to make fluids than to construct new cells. Consequently, there is a slight diminution of the density of the red cells which leads to the relative drop in the haemoglobin concentration of the woman's blood. It is to overcome this normal change that many women are given iron tablets in pregnancy.

During pregnancy you will notice your heart beating a lot more. You may have palpitations which you feel in the chest or in the throat. These are normal and merely a sign of the increased activity of the heart. Most healthy women have plenty of reserve in their heart and blood vessels to take the extra load of pregnancy and are in no way affected by it.

The lungs

All the oxygen you and your growing baby need is obtained through your lungs. Similarly, the waste gas carbon dioxide is excreted at that site. As the uterus increases in size it pushes the other contents of the stomach up under the diaphragm and so reduces the range of movements in the lower part of the lungs, for it is the diaphragm pulling down that usually increases chest size to cause air to enter the lungs. In pregnancy, diaphragmatic movements are impaired so that respiration depends more upon chest movements than upon the diaphragm. Generally, the total capacity of gas movement in and out of the chest is not decreased during pregnancy and you need not worry that you or your baby will be short of oxygen. It is merely that you will breathe in a different way and this becomes obvious in the middle months of pregnancy.

Urinary tract

One of the first changes you will notice in pregnancy is that you pass urine more frequently. This follows the release of hormones from the fetus, which influence the muscular wall of the bladder and so cause a mild irritation long before the growing uterus is big enough to press on the bladder itself. The

The mystery of pregnancy will enchant and delight other children in your family.

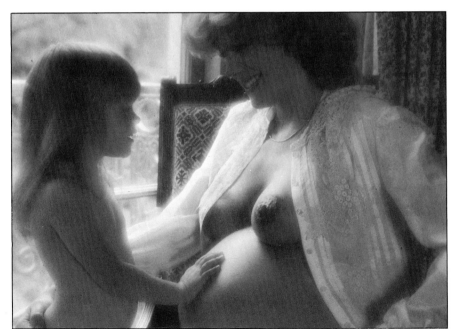

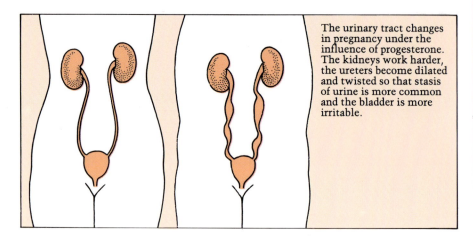

The urinary tract changes in pregnancy under the influence of progesterone. The kidneys work harder, the ureters become dilated and twisted so that stasis of urine is more common and the bladder is more irritable.

amount of urine passed during pregnancy is greater; the blood flow through each kidney is increased by up to 50 per cent so more water is filtered out of the blood. Normally, most of the water that leaves the body in the kidney via the collecting tubules is reabsorbed but, although in pregnancy the reabsorbtion rate increases, it cannot keep pace with the increase in water being filtered through the kidney. The tubes which connect the kidney to the bladder (the ureters) become slightly laxer in pregnancy under the influence of the same hormone, progesterone. Since these are fixed at each end, the result is that they become slightly convoluted and wider. Consequently, there is a hold-up of urine in them which leads to an increased rate of infection: whenever urine becomes stagnant it is an infection risk. This can be overcome by keeping a high fluid intake during pregnancy.

Digestive tract

HEARTBURN
In pregnancy, muscle guarding the lower end of the oesophagus is less strong; acid stomach juice flows back into the oesophagus and causes heartburn.

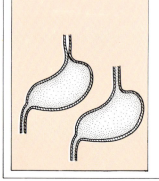

The organs concerned with the digestion of food and the extraction of nutrients are also affected by the pregnancy hormones. The intestine becomes less active and so a hold-up occurs, leading to the constipation that women commonly suffer during pregnancy. This can be relieved by increasing the quantity of high-fibre foods such as apples and bran.

There may be changes in the flow of fluids down the intestines so that reverse flow is more common. Some of the acid from the stomach may surge up into the gullet which is normally alkaline. This is felt as heartburn. Similarly, a reflux can occur from the intestine back to the stomach so that the alkaline contents enter what is normally an acid area; paradoxically, this is also noticed by the woman as pain in the upper stomach.

The liver, an organ that coordinates the regulation of hormones, acts less quickly and there is slower emptying of bile to the gallbladder.

These changes are perfectly normal and your body will soon get used to them. Only if they appear in an exaggerated form can they be called abnormal. If you have symptoms which concern you, you should discuss them with your doctor or midwife; they may be able to offer some treatment of the symptoms to relieve the worst excesses. The changes themselves, however, are within the normal range of behaviour of the normal mother-to-be and for these there is no treatment. You will have to put up with them and look forward to their disappearance after the birth of the baby.

GROWTH OF THE FETUS

During the three months of pregnancy from 14 to 27 weeks, fetal growth is very rapid. Growth occurs mostly by increasing the number of cells, the building blocks in the body. We all started when two cells fused — the egg from our mother and the sperm from our father. After this, growth is achieved by doubling the number of cells at each division. The divisions soon lead to some six billion cells in the fetus and the growth rate slows down. At 10 weeks all the organs are made and the fetus grows from a small human being into a larger one.

As soon as the limbs are formed, they start to move actively in the sac of fluid which encloses the fetus; because the fetal muscles are not very strong and because the walls of the uterus are thick, they probably have not yet been noticed by the mother. However, between 16 and 22 weeks of pregnancy most women will notice their baby moving inside the uterus. While the movements have been described as kicks, they are often felt more as flutters. To some women this is a very important time for it is the first real evidence that they have of a living being inside their body. These first movements cannot be pinned down to a precise date; some women feel them earlier than others. Those who have had a baby before and know what to expect will notice the movements earlier than women having their first baby. Generally speaking, most women who are having their first baby will have noticed movements by 20 weeks, though in subsequent pregnancies this can be brought forward by two or three weeks. There is little relationship between the movements felt at this stage of pregnancy and either the number of babies or the position in which the baby is lying. At this time there is plenty of fluid and the baby can move around like an aquatic mammal in a pool.

PILES
Piles are sometimes a problem in pregnancy; they are varicose veins just at the entrance to the anus and are caused by the increased pressure on the internal veins of the pelvis, due to the growing uterus. They are noticed either as soft purple lumps protruding through the anal ring or occasionally there is a little bright red bleeding if one of the bursts. They are a nuisance but do not usually have a serious effect and they get better after the baby has been born. They may be treated with cold compresses or local anaesthetic ointment that can be obtained from the chemist or the local antenatal clinic. Rarely is surgery required for piles during pregnancy.

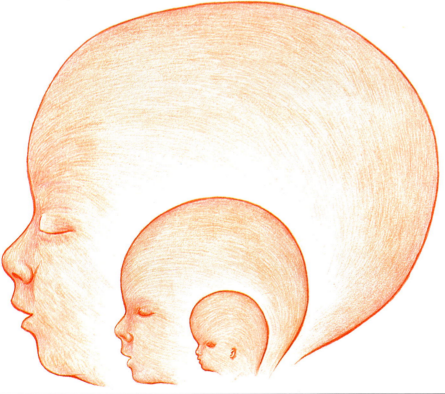

The fetal head is shown life-size at 10, 20 and 40 weeks. The rapid growth is mostly due to the increasing size of the brain.

The fetus grows throughout pregnancy but the production of amniotic fluid decreases towards the end (*right*). The fetus can no longer move so freely and remains fixed in position.

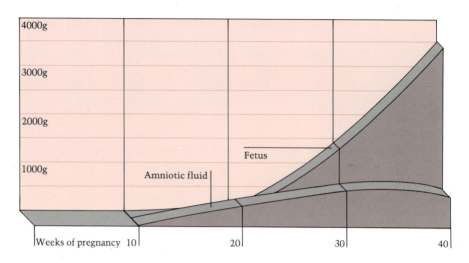

4000g

3000g

2000g

1000g

Fetus

Amniotic fluid

Weeks of pregnancy   10   20   30   40

The fetus can move round relatively freely in the middle of pregnancy. The amount of fluid allows him to present in these different ways (*right*) at 10.00 am, 2.00 pm and 7.00 pm in one day.

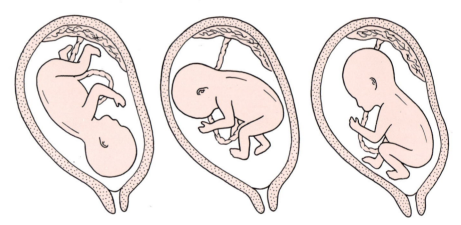

ANTENATAL INSTRUCTION

Preparation for childbirth is not just a matter of ensuring good physical care for you and your baby; you will need to prepare yourself physically and emotionally for this important event. The best way to do this is to arm yourself with as much reliable information as possible. If you know what is happening to you and why, you will be much better equipped to cope with the experience than someone for whom the situation is inexplicable and bewildering. Reading about pregnancy and childbirth is an invaluable basis for this preparation — but you should also try to attend antenatal classes where there is two-way communication, where you can put your questions to the professionals and talk to other women in the same situation.

There are different types of antenatal classes; they are mostly run by the local authority or hospital where you will deliver. (If you are having your baby at home you should still be able to attend classes at the local hospital — ask your midwife.) In addition the National Childbirth Trust (NCT) organizes classes on a local basis; you should contact the headquarters and they will put you in touch with your local organizer. It is important, for all types of classes, to find out early on in your pregnancy what is available in your area and to secure your place.

THE AIMS OF ANTENATAL CARE
● to prepare the mother physically for childbirth;
● to help the mother and her partner understand what is happening in childbirth and the time afterwards;
● to prepare the couple for the physical changes that are going to occur in the household with the newborn baby there.

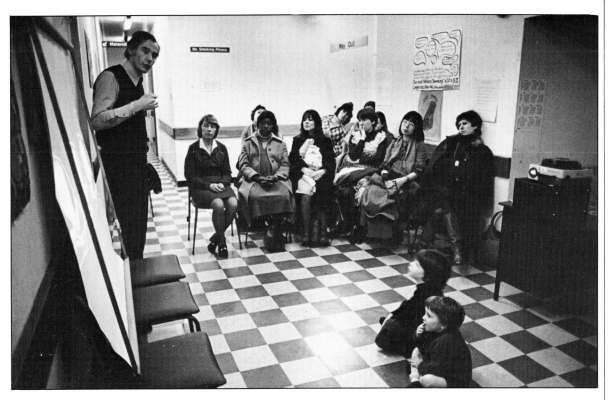

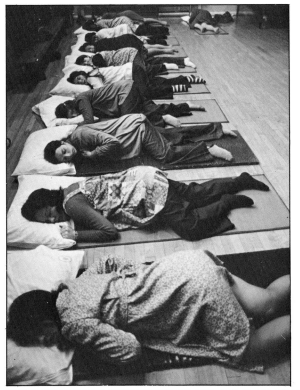

The doctor talking to a small group of women in a typical instructional class (*above*). Later, the mothers take part in relaxation exercises (*left*) in the physiotherapy department. Many women find benefit from more sophisticated exercises such as yoga (*below*). Do ensure that your instructor knows about your pregnancy and that your doctor knows about your yoga. All such exercises can be helpful depending upon the skill of the instructor.

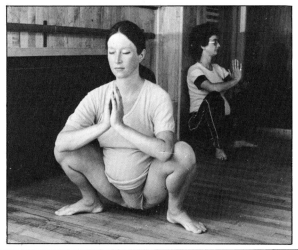

By strengthening your joints and ligaments these exercises may help you have a more comfortable pregnancy. None of these exercises is too strenuous, but take care not to overdo the routine.

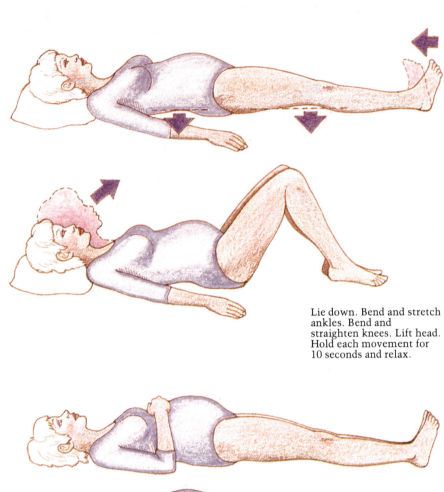

Lie down. Bend and stretch ankles. Bend and straighten knees. Lift head. Hold each movement for 10 seconds and relax.

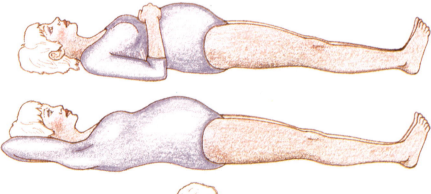

Squeeze buttocks together, tighten stomach muscles, press back and waist onto the floor. Hold for four seconds and relax.

Sit up straight. Tighten muscles around back passage for five seconds. Relax. Repeat four times.

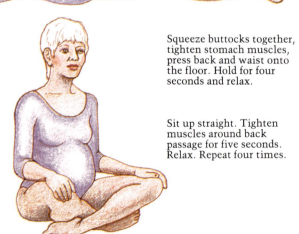

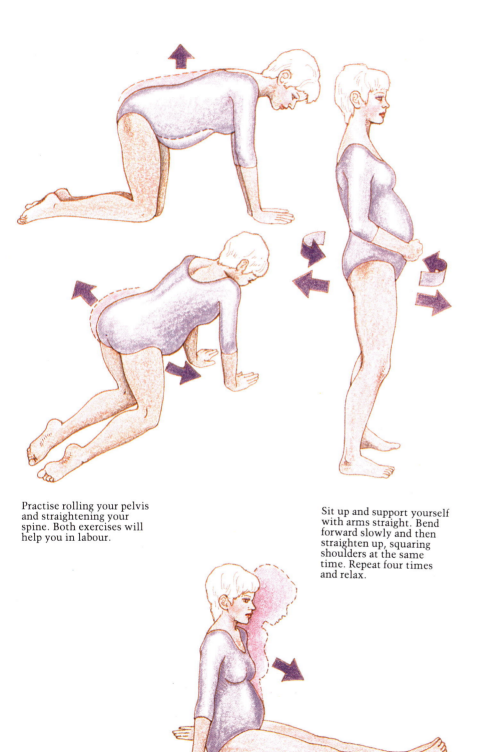

Practise rolling your pelvis and straightening your spine. Both exercises will help you in labour.

Sit up and support yourself with arms straight. Bend forward slowly and then straighten up, squaring shoulders at the same time. Repeat four times and relax.

The basis of most antenatal classes is instruction in the physical processes which take place during pregnancy and particularly in labour and childbirth. Many classes will then allow time for questions and discussion. Hospital classes will usually include a walk around the labour suites and the postnatal wards. Many classes end informally over a cup of tea so that you can chat to the other women. It is very often reassuring to discover during the informal part of the session that other women have fears and problems similar to yours. It is also a useful way of meeting women who are going to produce their babies at the same time as you; you will be able to make friends who will provide companionship and support during the early months when you are getting used to looking after your baby.

Some classes include exercises for childbirth. These are usually led by a trained physiotherapist and include limbering up and relaxation exercises. Finally there are group discussion classes which may be led by a midwife or NCT trained teacher. For these to be successful the groups have to be small and to meet regularly with a leader who is skilled at guiding the discussion unobtrusively.

The father's role

Your partner will want to be involved in this preparation for childbirth. Nearly all hospitals in the UK make fathers welcome in the delivery room, so it is best if he, like you, can learn as much as possible about what will happen there. He will be able to provide you with emotional support during the difficult patches and he may be able to provide physical support by rubbing your back or bringing you sips of water. Finally he will be there at the birth of his baby, an overwhelming experience and an immensely bonding process for all three of you.

At each visit to the antenatal clinic routine checks are carried out on your health and the development of the fetus. The results are recorded in the hospital notes and on a communication card, which is necessary if you are having shared-care with your GP.

PARTOGRAM

SPECIAL INSTRUCTIONS
PAEDIATRIC

OBSTETRIC

ANAESTHETIC   NAME LABEL

1.
2.
3.

TIME

DRUGS
EPIDURAL

Weak
Moderate
Strong

TIME

Fetal
Heart Rate
beats/min

LIQUOR
MOULDING
pH

C E R V I X

C E N T

LABOUR

CONDITION ON ADMISSION
DATE _____ TIME _____ GESTATION BY DATES _____
BY U/S _____
BP _____ PULSE _____ TEMP _____ URINE _____

MEMBRANES   INTACT/RUPTURED   TIME _____ DATE _____
LIQUOR   YES/NO   MECONIUM   YES/NO   FRESH/STALE
CONTRACTIONS   TIME OF ONSET ___ HR ___ DATE ___ REG/IRREG
FREQUENCY (PER 10 MINS) _____

FUNDAL HEIGHT _____ LIE _____ PRESENTATION & POSITION _____ P.PART ($^1/_5$) _____
F.H. _____ REG/IRREG _____

INDUCTION OF LABOUR   HR ___ DATE ___

INDICATION
METHOD
P.G. RIPENING _____ YES/NO
FORE/HIND ARM _____
SYNTOCINON _____ YES/NO

P.G. YES/NO ROUTE _____ DOSE _____
OTHER _____ DOSE _____

LIQUOR _____
INTERNAL / EXTERNAL   MONITOR
EPIDURAL/ ANALGESIA _____

BISHOP SCORE	Induction / Admission		
Cx.	0	1	2
Dilation (cm)	0	1 – 2	3 – 4
Consistency	FIRM	MEDIUM	SOFT
Length (cm)	> 2	1 – 2	< 1
Position	POSTERIOR	MID	ANTERIOR
Station	– 3	– 2	– 1.0
SCORE			

Labour progress is measured in hours rather than weeks. The lines of the partogram indicate the normal progress of many women having their first or subsequent babies. Dilatation of the cervix and descent of the baby's head are measured.

The time after delivery is important; midwives note the vital signs of temperature, pulse and the uterine size. If you go home early after delivery you take these notes with you.

PUERPERAL RECORDINGS

NUMBER _____

NAME

PUERPERIUM - ON DISCHARGE

GENERAL CONDITION _____   DATE _____
BREASTS _____   BP _____ URINE _____
ABDOMEN _____   Hb _____
UTERUS _____
VAGINAL EXAMINATION/PERINEUM _____
LOCHIA _____
FEEDING _____
SUGGESTED INVESTIGATIONS _____   POST NATAL VISIT FOR –
HOSPITAL _____
CONTRACEPTION ARRANGEMENTS _____   G.P. _____
LOCAL CLINIC _____
FUTURE PREGNANCY MANAGEMENT _____
DRUGS (T.T.A) _____
SIGN _____

HISTORY   POST NATAL VISIT
DATE _____
L.M.P _____
WEIGHT _____
BP _____
URINE _____

EXAMINATION
GENERAL _____   BREASTS _____
VAGINA _____   ABDOMEN _____
UTERUS _____   CERVIX _____
PERINEUM _____   DISCHARGE/BLEEDING _____
CYTOLOGY   DATE _____
RESULT _____
CONTRACEPTION –   CURRENT _____
FUTURE _____
REFERRAL TO OTHER DEPTS

Date
TIME
Temperature °C
Blood Pressure
Pulse
DAY
Lochia
Fundal Height (cm.)
Albumen

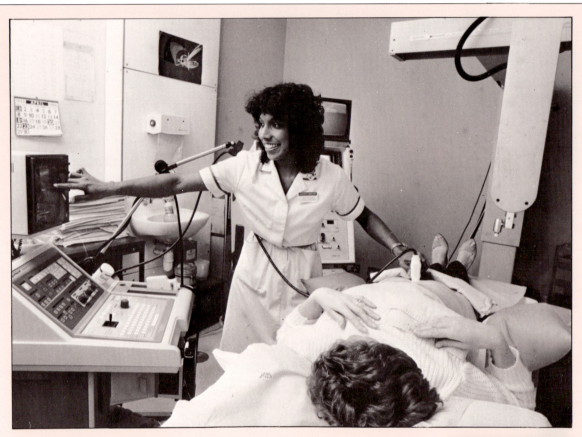

WHAT HAPPENS AT AN ULTRASOUND SCAN

During an ultrasound scan very small pulses of high-pitched sound waves are passed into the body and their echoes are collected as they bounce off hard objects. The transmitting source and the receiver are usually together in the head of the ultrasound machine.

You will be asked to lie down flat to have your scan and the ultrastenographer will usually wipe the front of your stomach with olive oil. This is to prevent any air getting trapped between the transmitting head and the skin, for air changes the sound waves' penetrating capacity. The head of the machine will then be passed over the abdomen in a series of arcs until the ultrastenographer has found the fetal parts to be measured: usually the fetal head. This will then

show up on the small visual display unit and you will be able to see your baby for the first time. In some departments where there is enough space, partners are invited in so they, too, can have the first glimpse of their child.

Ultrasound is a safe method of investigating the baby, for the dosage used is very small.

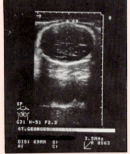

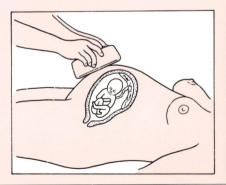

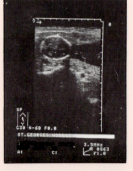

WORK IN PREGNANCY

The idea of a woman resting comfortably with someone bringing her a cup of tea every few hours is a very pleasant picture of the last months of pregnancy but it is now totally out of date. Nowadays most women continue their work into pregnancy and many work right up to the last moment (see also Chapter 1).

There is always work to be done in the home and this is in itself fatiguing, particularly if there are other children to be cared for. Meals have to be cooked, housework to be done and the general running of the home takes a lot of effort. If you work outside the home as well, then those tasks have to be squeezed into the early mornings, the evenings and weekends. Any woman who works in pregnancy should take extra care of herself. If you have to look after your home *and* your job you will probably have to sacrifice some of your social activities to make sure your body is not over-taxed in pregnancy.

At work make maximum use of any facilities which may be provided: rest rooms are there to be rested in. Talk to the occupational nurse if there is one at your workplace; she will be very sympathetic and guide you through early pregnancy, even acting as a buffer between you and your employers if necessary. Remember that you have the right to attend any antenatal clinics without loss of pay. Find out early on about the DHSS maternity grants and allowances and make sure that you get what you are entitled to.

If you enjoy your job and you are prepared to take sensible steps to make sure that you do not overstretch yourself, then there is no reason for you to give it up. Many women are so much more conscious of their body and its needs during pregnancy that they know when it is time to stop or reduce the level of work.

SOCIAL SECURITY BENEFITS

- Maternity Grant currently £25
  Claim from 14 weeks before, up to
  3 months after the birth.
- Maternity Allowance currently
  £25.95 per week.
  Payable for 18 weeks starting from
  11 weeks before the baby is due.
  Entitlement depends on National
  Insurance contributions. Claim 14
  weeks before baby is due.
- Prescriptions and dental treatment
  Free during pregnancy and for one
  year after the birth.
- Milk and vitamins
  If you are claiming Supplementary
  Benefit, you will be entitled to
  free milk and vitamins.

- Child Benefit currently £6.50 per
  week
  Payable to all mothers in respect
  of each child.
- One Parent Benefit currently
  £4.05 per week
  Payable to single parents for the
  first child and in addition to child
  benefit.

Claims forms for these benefits can be obtained from your GP or local social security office.

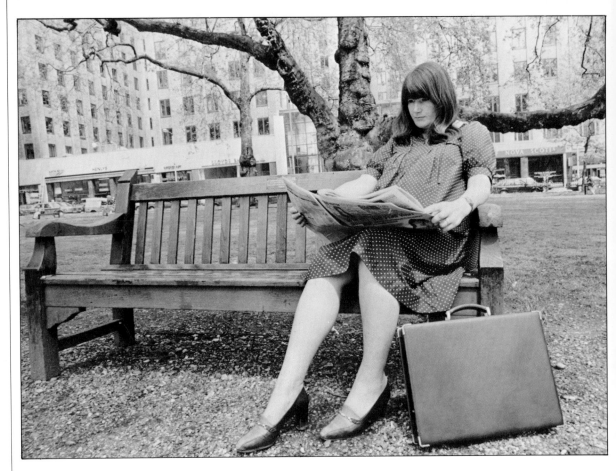

Take advantage of your lunch breaks to relax — you need all the rest you can get at this stage.

DIET

Remember to maintain a healthy diet even if your appetite wanes. The principles outlined in Chapter 1 should be followed throughout pregnancy.

ABNORMAL DEVELOPMENT

The most common of the serious fetal abnormalities occur due to an error in development inside the uterus. Many organs of the body are made by the fusion of tubes or the breaking down of partitions between two tubes. If the normal pattern of events in the baby's body is disturbed in very early pregnancy abnormalities can occur. The less serious of these are dealt with on pages 170 to 171.

Disturbances from outside the fetal body which affect fusion can be of various sorts. They may be due to irradiation (if a woman has had a series of X-rays of the lower abdomen, not knowing she was pregnant) or to drugs (the best known example was thalidomide, discovered to be a drug dangerous to the fetal development in the early 1960s). A wide series of other, less specific hazards exist that may affect the fetus and of which the mother is not aware at the time. One of the major problems in spotting developmental abnormalities is that they are caused before the woman realizes she is pregnant, in the first five or six weeks after fertilization.

It is impossible to check an unborn fetus for every congenital abnormality, but some of the major ones can be detected early and the parents advised so that action may be taken. There may be a family history of conditions like haemophilia or dwarfism and, in such cases, the risks to a couple can be determined by expert genetic counselling. Thus they can know of the possibility of this problem occurring. Similarly, the probability of conditions like cystic fibrosis and thalassaemia can be determined on a risk basis by examination of the family tree. These are minority diseases; the real use of antenatal fetal screening is in the detection of two more common conditions. One is a chromosomally determined state, Down's Syndrome, the other is a defect in fusion of the nervous system tube which results in a group of open central nervous system abnormalities such as anencephaly and spina bifida.

Screening for disease

MAJOR MALFORMATIONS
Per 100,000 live births

CENTRAL NERVOUS SYSTEM		GASTROINTESTINAL	
Microcephaly (small head)	16	Inguinal hernia	1-30
Hydrocephaly (water on the brain)	14	Pyloric stenosis (funtional obstruction to stomach outflow)	19
Spina bifida	7	Umbilical hernia	12
Anencephaly (absence of brain)	6	Cleft palate	11
MUSCULO-SKELETAL SYSTEM		Hare lip	11
Talipes (club feet)	69		
Hip instability or dislocation	43	GENITOURINARY SYSTEM	
Wryneck	13	Hypospadias (undescended testicles) — both sides	18
Scoliosis and kyphosis (curvature of the spine)	7	Hydroureter (dammed-back urine)	8
Fingers missing	5	Cystic kidneys	6
Toes missing	5		
CARDIORESPIRATORY SYSTEM		OTHER SYSTEMS	
Underdevelopment of lung	13	Cavernous haemangioma (birth marks)	70
Ventricular septal defect (hole in heart)	11	Down's Syndrome (mongolism)	11
Atrial septal defect (hole in heart)	5	Congenital cataract (one cause of blindness)	9
Patent ductus arteriosis (persistent bypass)	8		

Down's Syndrome

Down's Syndrome or mongolism occurs in about 1 in 600 births. It is rarely fatal unless accompanied by other abnormalities of the heart or intestines; the child is usually physically normal but mentally subnormal. It is well known to happen more frequently in older mothers (aged 35 and more) and the risks increase rapidly after the age of 40. Although the risk is less in younger women, the number of such women having babies is much greater and so it occurs in appreciable numbers even in the youngest age group. All the chromosomes in each cell of the body are the same and they can be teased out of their tangled skein and grouped into 23 pairs. These pairs of chromosomes are designated by the numbers 1 to 23. When cell division occurs in the ovary or testis, one of each of these pairs goes into the egg or the sperm. Occasionally, and increasingly with age, both the chromosomes of a group go together. Hence, if this happens in the ovary, an egg is made with two 23 chromosomes and when this is fertilized with a sperm with its own 23rd chromosome, there will be three chromosomes at position 23, thus a trisomy will be made.

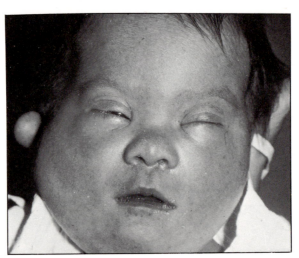

Down's Syndrome (Mongolism) is responsible for about a third of mental retardation in infants. Babies with this condition can be recognized by characteristic signs of slit eyes, wide nose and low-set ears.

Number of babies with Down's syndrome

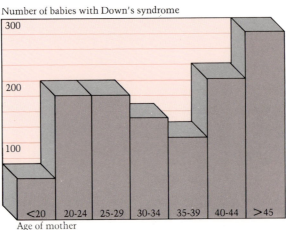

Age of mother

The risk of Down's Syndrome is greater for a woman in the older age group. However, the number of young women having babies is much greater and so a considerable number of Down's syndrome babies is produced even in the younger age group.

The antenatal detection of babies with Down's Syndrome depends upon getting some of the cells from the fetus so that the chromosome content of the nuclei can be checked. The best way of doing this is by amniocentesis — the removal of some of the fluid around the baby. Into the fluid have been shed fetal skin cells containing the same chromosome constitution as all the other cells of the body. Unfortunately there is not a high enough concentration of these skin cells until after the 16th week of pregnancy and so amniocentesis is usually done between 16 and 18 weeks of gestation. A small sample of fluid is removed from around the fetus under local anaesthetic. This is spun down to get a high concentration of fetal cells from the sediment and the cells are cultured for 20 days. The nuclei of the cells are then examined and the chromosome patterns can be determined.

Usually this test is very specific and in most cases shows clearly whether the baby has or has not got a chromosome abnormality. If the chromosomes do show a trisomy then the couple will be advised about the future. The only medical treatment that can be offered is a termination of pregnancy. Because

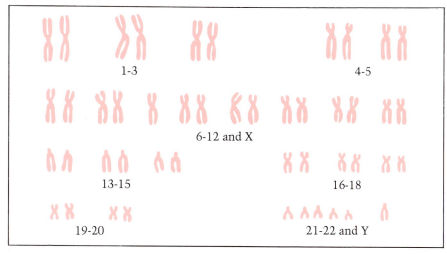

Chromosome pattern showing fetal cells with a trisomy — a positive result in testing for Down's Syndrome (above).

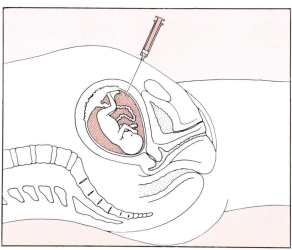

Removal of the fluid from around the baby allows the chemical content of the fluid and the cells shed by the fetus to be examined. It is not a painful procedure.

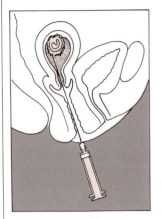

Tissue containing genetic material from the fetus can be removed in early pregnancy so that, after culture, the chromosome make-up of the unborn child can be determined.

of the time needed to grow the cells, it is obvious that 19 to 20 weeks of pregnancy will have passed before a result is available. An abortion at this stage is much more difficult than one earlier on but many couples prefer this rather than to give birth to a child with Down's Syndrome.

More recently, techniques have been developed which take a small sample of the fetal cells much earlier. At about eight weeks of pregnancy the cells around the growing embryo sac start to retreat so that a lesser number of them become the placenta. A minute tube may be passed through the cervix and manoeuvred up into these cells, allowing a small sample to be taken without disturbing the growing embryo. These cells may be cultured so that knowledge of their chromosomal content is obtained by 11 or 12 weeks of gestation, a time which makes recommendations for therapeutic intervention in the pregnancy much easier. At present this method, known as chorionic biopsy, is experimental and is carried out in only half a dozen centres in the UK, but it is probable that in the next five years it will become more uniformly available and with it earlier termination of pregnancy will be more acceptable.

There is an additional problem with amniocentesis, for passing a needle into the amniotic sac carries a very small risk. This risk is probably less than one per cent but the procedure may stimulate the muscle and cause the uterus to contract; this results in an abortion at 16 weeks, obviously an undesirable event if the fetus is normal. Consequently doctors are loath to offer amniocentesis unless there are good grounds for it. If you look at the risk chart for age of mother in relation to Down's Syndrome, it is obvious that a woman of 30 has such a low risk of producing a baby with Down's Syndrome that there would be approximately an eight to ten times greater chance of harming a normal baby by amniocentesis than of diagnosing a baby with Down's Syndrome. Conversely, by the age of 40 the risks of detecting the condition (about one per cent) are about the same as the risks of the side effects to amniocentesis. Consequently, the policy now is to offer all women over 40 years amniocentesis; any woman between 35 and 40 who wishes it can usually get an amniocentesis fairly readily. For the reasons explained here, most obstetricians would advise women under 35 not to have this test.

Open central nervous system abnormalities

You have seen on page 32 how a ridge of skin sinks into the back and folds close over it to produce a hollow tube which becomes the brain and the spinal cord. Occasionally, in the early weeks of pregnancy something happens to prevent the ridges from closing and so an opening is left. The most common sites for this are either in the lower back or in the head so that nervous tissue is left exposed. Thus the brain or spinal cord is exposed and infection could easily occur. Spina bifida is not automatically a fatal condition but unfortunately two-thirds of babies with an open spina bifida do not live beyond one month, despite surgery which can be done to close the defect. Anencephaly, on the other hand, is inevitably a fatal condition. Without a brain the body cannot survive outside the uterus and no anencephalic survives more than an hour or two; many are born dead. With these bad prognoses, many couples would not wish to continue the pregnancy of a fetus with an open neural tube defect, if they knew about it in time to choose an abortion.

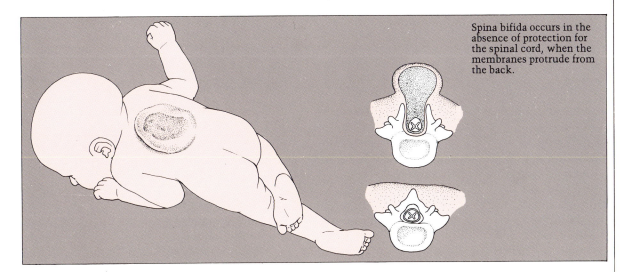

Spina bifida occurs in the absence of protection for the spinal cord, when the membranes protrude from the back.

The open lining of the neural tube in both spina bifida and anencephaly allows the leakage into the mother's blood stream of a chemical made by the fetus. This is alpha fetoprotein which can be detected fairly easily. Unfortunately, the concentrations of this protein do not rise early in pregnancy and so the test cannot be performed until about 16 to 18 weeks of gestation. A blood test done on the mother at this time may detect a raised level. If this is confirmed by a second blood test, the couple will usually be advised to undergo amniocentesis in order to check the level of alpha fetoprotein in the fluid surrounding the baby in the uterus. The procedure is the same as the amniocentesis already described, but the chemical test on the fluid is much quicker and a result is usually known within two or three days. If this, too, shows a raised level the couple may be advised about a termination of pregnancy.

There is no chemical test which can be carried out earlier than the alpha fetoprotein test at 16 weeks but, in some centres, the skill of doctors using ultrasound has increased so much that the defect in the bony spinal column which accompanies spina bifida can be seen at about 15 or 16 weeks. Similarly, the absence of head bones may be detected at this time and so anencephaly can be diagnosed. It is possible in the next few years that the more frequent use of ultrasound and the greater skills of those using it may lead to a diminution of the use of alpha fetoprotein testing and an increase in ultrasound testing for spina bifida and anencepahaly. Unfortunately, the treatment to be offered is still the same; one can only offer to stop the pregnancy.

Unlike Down's Syndrome, there is no particular age group of mothers who produce babies with abnormalities of the spinal cord and brain. There are very few ways one can make the diagnosis of higher risk and so the only way to detect such a fetus in the uterus would be to offer a blood test for alpha fetoprotein (or a special ultrasound test) to all pregnant women. In areas where there is a higher risk of these conditions, this is already being done. The problem is that in areas where the incidence is lower than 1 in 1,000 women, it becomes difficult to maintain a screening service.

Screening

There are other rarer conditions detectable in the antenatal period. Some of the other chromosome conditions can be diagnosed by examination of the amniotic fluid. At present, special tests are being done to examine the protein enzymes which the fetus produces, in an effort to make an earlier diagnosis of cystic fibrosis. Some conditions (such as thalassaemia) which can be spotted by examination of the fetal blood are now being diagnosed in the uterus by passing a fetoscope through into the amniotic fluid and then directly drawing a sample of the fetal blood from the arteries and veins as they course over the placental surface. In addition, ultrasound is becoming more precise and some congenital abnormalities of the kidneys and heart can be diagnosed precisely by careful skilled ultrasound. These are all, however, very special tests which need a lot of time and resources and they are carried out at very few centres at present. If the obstetrician thinks that the fetus has got a chance of having any other rarer conditions, the mother will probably be referred to one of these special centres.

The checks for Down's Syndrome among older women, and for abnormalities of the central nervous system, can be offered as a screening service to women attending any hospital which performs antenatal care. One of the most important results from using such a screening service is that, in the vast majority of cases, the obstetrician can tell the mother in the middle of her pregnancy that she is carrying a normal child. If a woman has previously had an abnormality of this nature and she can be told early on, long before delivery, that her unborn child is normal; this is an immensely important aspect of the care of that woman in pregnancy. It not only leads to obvious happiness and relief but to a much healthier woman who approaches labour in a very different frame of mind. It is a most important part of medicine to be able to relieve anxiety.

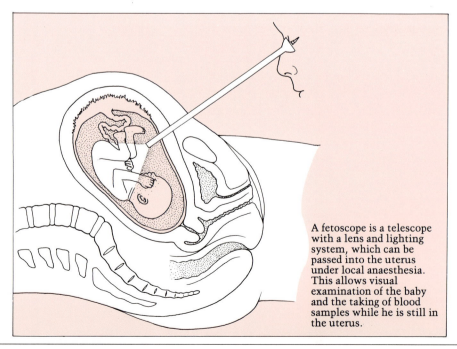

A fetoscope is a telescope with a lens and lighting system, which can be passed into the uterus under local anaesthesia. This allows visual examination of the baby and the taking of blood samples while he is still in the uterus.

PROBLEMS OF PREGNANCY

Most women go through their pregnancy without any problems. A few, however, do suffer from conditions specific to pregnancy. Most of these start later on so will be dealt with in the next section but one condition can be detected early and needs early management — the rhesus problem.

Rhesus problem

By contrast with many other species, the human has evolved so that members are distinguished one from the other by having blood of different groups. If these are mixed, the blood is destroyed and serious consequences ensue. If a blood transfusion is needed, the donor blood will be carefully checked to be of the same group as the recipient. The most common blood groups are A, B, AB and O; and it is to the last group that most people's blood belongs. Independent of this system, and unrelated to it, is the distinction of blood into two other categories, rhesus-positive and rhesus-negative. Rhesus refers to the difference in these two types of blood first noted as a result of research with the rhesus monkey. Eighty-five per cent of the population of Britain are rhesus-positive but 15 per cent are rhesus-negative for they have no rhesus antigens. Other countries have a much smaller proportion of rhesus-negative people.

The rhesus-negative gene is a recessive one and, as shown earlier, this means that the baby will only be rhesus-negative if he receives chromosomal material with rhesus-negative genes from both father and mother. Should only one parent pass a gene, the baby will be rhesus-positive but would be a carrier, ie he or she could produce children if mated with a rhesus-negative partner. Outside pregnancy, the rhesus condition is rarely a problem. Anyone who is going to have a blood transfusion is cross matched for the rhesus factor and so no trouble ensues. However, in pregnancy there may be a problem if the blood of the fetus inside the uterus is a different rhesus group from that of the mother. Obviously if the mother is rhesus-positive, she can only carry a rhesus-positive fetus for the gene is recessive. If, however, the mother is rhesus-negative she may be carrying a rhesus-negative baby (should she, by

The proportion of rhesus-negative people differs in different parts of the world. The proportion of 15 per cent seen in Western Europe is high; it is much less in the Middle and Far East, dropping to 3 per cent in parts of the Far East.

Rhesus family

Rhesus state of parents

Homozygos   Heterozygos

Rhesus state of offspring

It is only when a rhesus-positive father and a rhesus-negative mother come together that a rhesus-negative mother can be carrying a rhesus-positive baby; even then the risk of one having an effect on the other is only 1 in 200.

chance have a rhesus-negative partner) or one who is rhesus-positive. In the former instance there is no problem but the latter may give rise to difficulties.

It sometimes happens that a few fetal blood cells escape across the placenta and enter the mother's bloodstream. If these should be rhesus-positive and the mother rhesus-negative, they would act as a foreign protein and stimulate the formation of antibodies in the mother's blood. This particular reaction would not harm the mother with the small amount of fetal red cells that leak across. She is rhesus-negative and the antibody is only lethal to rhesus-positive red cells. However, these antibodies can diffuse back through the placental membrane into the baby's circulation. Here, being rhesus antibodies, they attack fetal rhesus-positive blood cells, destroying them and releasing their contents. If this reaction were to go on long enough, the fetus would become anaemic and the breakdown products of the haemoglobin would collect in the tissues. These are toxic and may affect vital brain centres producing neurological symptoms.

The rhesus condition becomes a problem in about 1 in every 200 deliveries. All women in early pregnancy have their rhesus group checked at the first antenatal visit. If it is positive then there is no further problem. Should however the woman be rhesus-negative, she is then checked to see if any antibodies develop in pregnancy. It is very rare for such a leak to occur before mid-pregnancy; it takes some six to eight weeks for antibody reaction to occur after a leak. The major time for sensitization usually occurs during separation of the placenta after the baby's birth and so it is too late to affect that particular baby. This can however act as a stimulus to a future antibody formation. The first tests for antibodies on a rhesus-negative mother are made at the booking visit. If they are negative, they are repeated at 30 weeks and again at about 36 weeks. When the rhesus-negative woman becomes pregnant for the second time, if she bears a rhesus-positive infant again, some of the fetal red cells may go across to her circulation in mid-pregnancy and a brisk

If a rhesus positive baby is carried by a rhesus negative mother (1), sensitization can occur at delivery (2). In subsequent pregnancies (3), another rhesus positive fetus may be affected by the antibodies made by the mother (4).

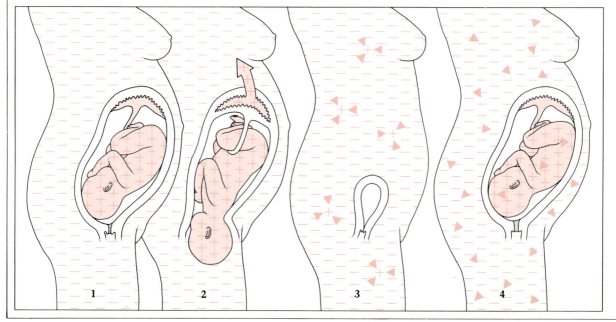

response then occurs. Antibodies are made rapidly, for the antibody-forming tissue has been previously sensitized. The antibodies pass back across the placenta and may affect the baby. Consequently, the blood checks of a rhesus-negative woman having her second or third baby are more rigorous than of one having her first.

The degree of fetal effect relates approximately to the level of antibodies. If there is a higher concentration, there is a greater risk that the unborn baby will be affected. To specify these risks more carefully, fluid is taken from around the baby by amniocentesis and examined for the breakdown products of haemoglobin. If these are raised, a more precise risk to the fetus can be determined. The ultimate treatment of the rhesus-affected fetus is to remove him from the noxious surroundings of antibodies pouring across the placenta and, if necessary, to perform an exchange transfusion in the neonatal nursery to wash out such antibodies present in his blood. Until 20 years ago this was all we had to offer. It often meant inducing babies who were very immature and who were at great risk of suffering from their lack of maturity as well as their rhesus problem. More recently, two advances have improved the situation.

1 Intrauterine transfusions

Under ultrasound control and local anaesthesia, a soft plastic catheter is passed through the mother's stomach wall, through the uterine wall, across the amniotic fluid and into the abdominal cavity of the fetus. Through this a small transfusion of rhesus-negative blood is given to top up the baby's own blood supply and allow him to stay in the uterus a week or two longer. This allows a greater maturity to be achieved if induction is needed. Such an intrauterine transfusion staves off anaemia for a week or two but it may have to be repeated.

2 Blocking serum

An even more hopeful line of treatment has been developed in Britain and America and is now applied almost universally in the West. The time when most fetal red cells go across the placenta to stimulate antigen formation is at the delivery of the placenta. Injection of a blocking serum, consisting of modified antibodies, can be given to prevent the action of the stimulating factor. These modified antibodies to the rhesus-positive factor will not last long enough to affect any child of a subsequent pregnancy, but will prevent the woman's body from making her own. If this treatment is correctly applied, a rhesus-negative woman thus approaches each pregnancy as though it were her first, a time of minimal risk. Treatment with anti-D-gamma-globulin is now universally applied and any woman who is rhesus-negative and has produced a rhesus-positive baby is usually given the injection within 48 hours of birth.

The use of this preventative therapy has revolutionized the management of the rhesus condition and it is now much less common to see affected babies in Western society. It does have the disadvantage, however, that when such babies do occur there are fewer centres that are skilled to deal with them and the mother may have to travel some distance in order to get good treatment and ensure that her unborn fetus has the best chance of survival. Overcoming the rhesus problem is, however, one of the major triumphs of antenatal care in the last 20 years and has almost eliminated the rhesus problem in the UK.

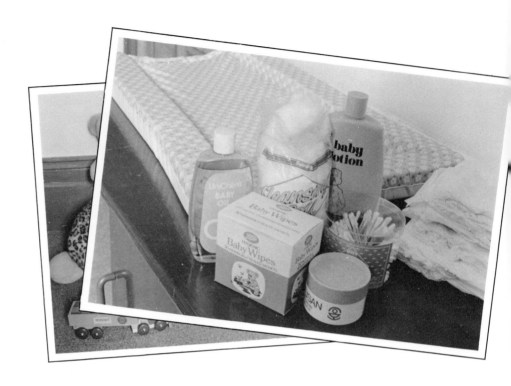

THE LATE MONTHS

By 28 weeks of gestation a baby weighs about 1 kg. If he was born at this stage he would be immature and have difficulty in surviving. If labour were to start it would be wise for the mother to go urgently to a special obstetrics department attached to a Special Care Baby Unit used to dealing with small babies. In such a unit, a baby of this size would stand a 75 per cent chance of doing well, but if the baby was delivered in an ordinary hospital without special neonatal facilities, that chance would drop to 50 per cent. As the weeks go by, the child develops fast so that by 32 weeks of gestation the birthweight might be expected to be 1.5 kg and by 36 weeks 2.5 kg. Survival rates improve rapidly as maturity of the fetus is established.

The amount of fluid around the baby is increasing during this time so that there is on average about 0.5 l at 28 weeks rising to about 1 to 1.5 l by 40 weeks. At this stage of pregnancy, the fluid is made mostly from fetal urine; his kidneys are working and he passes urine through his bladder into his private swimming pool. The rest of the fluid is made by the passage of water from the mother's blood circulating in the membranes which make up the sac surrounding the baby. The position the fetus takes in his mother's uterus at 28 weeks gestation is not constant. The volume of fluid is high by comparison with the size of the body of the baby, so he can float into any position. After 32 weeks of pregnancy he tends to grow at a slightly faster rate than the fluid is produced and so relatively occupies more space. By this time he is usually lying vertically in the uterus with his head at the lower end. This is not caused by gravity — it is the best way for the baby to fit into the uterus. The bunched up feet against the buttocks are wider than the fetal head so they fit into the broader upper end of the uterus better than does the head, which finds its place at the narrower lower end. By 36 weeks, most babies have achieved their final position which is usually lying longitudinally in the uterus with the head presenting. About three per cent of babies, however, will be longitudinal with the buttocks presenting (breech presentation) and about one per cent will be lying transversely.

A transverse position is difficult, for it is not possible to deliver a woman vaginally of a baby who is lying persistently at right angles to the exit and so he is potentially at risk. Should the baby stay in this position the woman would be admitted to hospital so that attempts could be made to move him into the longitudinal position; this can be done by gentle manipulation through the mother's abdominal wall.

After about 36 weeks, the volume of amniotic fluid diminishes slightly so that the fetus fills the uterus even more tightly. At the same time the head often engages into the pelvis and you will notice a lightening of the load in your stomach. As the fetal head goes down past the entrance to the pelvis it is said to engage and you will notice this by the lower position of the whole fetus in your abdomen; you will have a little more space at the top end for your stomach to expand.

Engagement of the fetal head into the pelvis has important obstetrical implications. If the fetal head passes into the pelvis there is a 95 per cent chance of a vaginal delivery. Conversely, if a head will not engage in the pelvis, this is a sign that there may be some disproportion between the size of that baby and the mother; the doctor will pay particular attention to this to see if the baby can be helped to engage. If not, it may be that that particular baby is too big for that particular pelvis and a Caesarian section may be required to deliver the baby. This is one of the important signs looked for in the last weeks of pregnancy. With the diminution in the relative volume of liquor, the obstetrician can feel the baby more readily through the abdominal wall, so that he can tell where the shoulders, the back and the limbs are.

The reduction in volume of amniotic fluid means that your total weight gain in the latter weeks of pregnancy may be reduced or even stopped. This is not serious and happens to most women. The fluid surrounding the baby is constantly being produced and absorbed so that a steady state is reached when the rates of production and reabsorption equal each other. Occasionally this balance is disturbed. If more is made than absorbed, then an excess of fluid occurs. This is called polyhydramnios. The excess fluid allows the baby to float around too freely and this may give rise to abnormal presentations in later pregnancy, for his head may not engage in the pelvis. This is a very uncomfortable condition and the uterus is very stretched and sore. Admission to hospital may be necessary and diuretics may be needed to reduce the amount of fluid in the body. Occasionally, fluid accumulates so

The fetus is shown at 28 (*right*) and at 40 weeks (*centre*) of pregnancy. At 28 weeks the proportion of fluid is much greater so that he can move around. By 40 weeks there is relatively little fluid and he is fixed in one of several possible positions (*far right*).

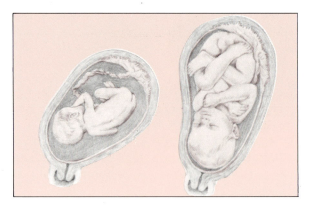

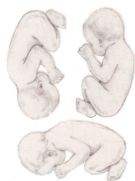

fast that it is very painful and needs to be drained, but this is uncommon. The converse is when less fluid is made than is being reabsorbed, so there is a lack of fluid—oligohydramnios—and the baby is compressed by the uterine sac. A lack of fluid is not a good sign, it is often associated with slower growth of the fetus who is pinched inside the tightly-fitting uterine sac.

Commonly, the membranes surrounding the fetus are maintained intact until halfway through labour. When the cervix is dilating the membranes burst and some fluid escapes. Occasionally, however, the cervix of the womb is not as strong as it should be and a little bulge of membranes passes down into the cervical canal. This allows for a weak point in the bag of membranes which may burst prematurely causing the amniotic fluid to leak out. Such an event is often followed by uterine contractions so that a pre-term labour follows with a baby who is smaller than expected. This is unusual and 98 per cent of labours start after the 34th week of pregnancy when the baby is more mature and able to survive in the outside world.

WHAT TO DO IN THE LAST WEEKS

Many women stop work by about 28 weeks of pregnancy. This is when you may become entitled to maternity benefit and it also corresponds with the time that many women start to feel bulky and uncomfortable. Many find that being forced to remove themselves from the workplace does not make a holiday, however. There is often more than enough to do at home, so, despite having given up work, you may be more tired at this stage. Of course, there is a

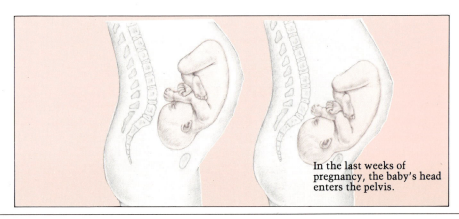

In the last weeks of pregnancy, the baby's head enters the pelvis.

larger load of baby and uterus to carry around; this disturbs the equilibrium of the body so that you tend to arch your back more and make use of muscles you would not be using normally.

Try to accept that the load of pregnancy is at its greatest in the last phase and rest more. Ideally you should rest properly in bed for at least an hour every afternoon as well as going to bed earlier and getting up later. If there are other children in the family this can be difficult; try to enlist the help of family and friends to give you time to rest. Late pregnancy is not a time for moving or redecorating your present home. Do not take on any extra non-essential tasks. Your partner should help with the housework, shopping and care of other children as much as possible. You will need emotional support, too, at this time; if your partner has attended some antenatal classes with you, he will feel more involved in the pregnancy and more understanding of the problems.

Intercourse can continue for as long as you wish or for as long as your ingenuity finds ways to overcome the obstacles. The growing lump in the front of the stomach makes the conventional missionary position difficult. However, if you wish, other positions can be equally pleasurable well into late pregnancy. The woman may wish to be the dominant partner and be on top, or entry may be from the rear. There are many myths about the hazards of intercourse in late pregnancy. It has been said to cause infection in the uterus or that it may start off labour prematurely. Neither of these claims can be substantiated and there is no reason why you should not behave as you wish.

BACK ACHE

By standing upright, our species has put a strain on the lower back. In pregnancy there is an increase in hormone levels which leads to a softening of the ligaments guarding the lumber vertebrae and the junction of the sacrum with the pelvic bones. The increasing load of the uterus causes the back to arch more and so any weakness will show up. As the baby grows in the last weeks of pregnanoy and his head enters the pelvis, this too puts pressure on the nerves at the back of the pelvis and can cause backache.

If you have had back problems prior to pregnancy, these may be exacerbated now. You should avoid heavy tasks and, while moderate exercise is sensible, moving the furniture or gardening may produce problems. The best treatment in pregnancy is bedrest with firm support to the spine. Should the backache be on one side it often helps to lie on the other side so that the fetal presenting part is not pressing on any nerves. Many women find that heat from a hot water bottle is helpful, and the use of pain-relieving drugs is usually safe, but they should be discussed with your doctor as should the use of any muscle-relaxing drugs.

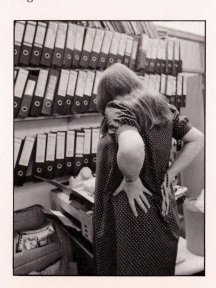

As the fetus and the uterus grow, they compress the normal contents of the abdomen above and behind them. Pregnancy causes the front wall of the abdomen to be stretched. The stomach and intestines all have to be kept behind the growing uterus in the back of the abdomen.

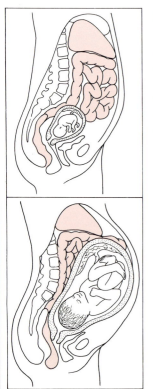

The increased physical burden of late pregnancy often means that desire is lessened and many couples may give up intercourse at this time, but there is no medical reason for this. Of course, sexual pleasure does not need to be confined to intercourse and many couples find this a good opportunity to find other ways of giving and gaining physical pleasure.

In later pregnancy, you may feel you do not wish to eat so much. The increasing mass of the uterus is pressing the stomach and intestines considerably to the back of the stomach cavity. However, the nutritional needs of the mother and baby still need to be maintained and so it is probably wise to have a series of small, but pleasantly nutritious meals throughout the day. Rather than a formal breakfast, lunch and supper, it would be better to have a light breakfast, a mid-morning snack, lunch, tea, light supper and a small snack before going to bed. This does not mean you should overeat, rather that the protein and energy requirements should be spread more evenly through the day so that no extra physical load is put upon the stomach during this time of compression. Some women find, with approaching labour, that their appetite decreases; this varies from woman to woman.

ANTENATAL CARE

As pregnancy advances, antenatal visits become more frequent. Having been monthly up to this time, they now become fortnightly and, after 36 weeks, weekly. This may seem a terrible chore to someone who is feeling perfectly well. The journey to the hospital, the sitting around waiting, the brief time with the doctor or midwife and then the long journey back—all are burdensome, especially if you have to take other children with you. However, it is during this phase of antenatal care that your medical and midwifery advisers can spot problems and it is now that antenatal care is at its most acute and useful.

By 30 weeks, a multiple pregnancy (twins or more) will have been diagnosed in most women. With the recently increased use of ultrasound, the diagnosis may well have been made very much earlier in pregnancy, but clinical diagnoses are not usually made until after the 26th week. Blood tests for anaemia and a check for antibodies of those women who are rhesus-negative will be made around this time.

In the ensuing weeks of pregnancy, the growth of the fetus will be monitored carefully by the examining obstetricians and midwives. As the weeks go by, he can be felt more clearly through the uterus so that the experienced doctor or midwife can tell where he is lying; they can find his head, his back and his buttocks and thus can relate the lie of the baby to the mother. It is important that he lies in a longitudinal axis for this is the way that most babies will deliver. The vast majority (96 per cent) will end up with their head in the pelvis and their buttocks at the top end of the uterus, in the manner described earlier.

At each visit, you will be checked for your general fitness and any symptoms that may have arisen will be discussed. Your blood pressure, weight and urine will all be checked. After 36 weeks all this antenatal effort is intensified to a weekly visit to ensure that the head engages, as has been described, and that the baby is growing sensibly. In many hospitals, at this

RAISED BLOOD PRESSURE.

The degree of rise in blood pressure seen in most women during pregnancy is quite mild compared with the hypertension that general physicians look after in later life. It is rare for the woman herself to suffer from this raised pressure, for her kidneys, heart and brain blood vessels can stand the slight increase. If the raised pressure were to persist it could lead to a condition of fitting but this is very rare.

More commonly the rise in pressure is associated with a poorer perfusion of the placental bed so that the fetus suffers from undernutrition.

stage, the pelvis will be examined by an internal assessment. You may not find this very pleasant but it is an essential part of the assessment of the inter-relationship between the fetus and the mother. The head of the baby should be engaged in the pelvis in the last weeks of pregnancy and the cervix should be ripening. This is all checked by a simple internal vaginal examination. If the head of the fetus does not engage, it is even more essential that an internal examination is carried out to see if there is a disproportion between the size of the baby's head and the size of the mother's pelvis.

Most women deliver around the time of the expected date of delivery. A few, however, go on after this date. If this happens, try not to be disappointed — the estimated date of delivery is only a mathematical probability, not a certainty. Unless there is a medical complication which presses for immediate delivery no action will be taken by the obstetrician. In many cases, the woman is asked to come back to the antenatal clinic one week later; some will not make this appointment for they will have gone into labour spontaneously before then. Those who do turn up at 41 weeks will be assessed carefully to see how much further into pregnancy it will be safe to allow them to proceed. For some, another weekly appointment will be given; for others, induction before the 42nd week will be considered. The obstetrician and the woman concerned will have to discuss this together. There is statistical evidence to show that if a baby passes 42 weeks there is much greater danger of a difficult and possibly damaging delivery. The placenta has a limited lifespan and is probably at its functional best for transferring nutrients and oxygen to the baby at about 37 weeks. From then on it starts to age and its function gets slightly less efficient each week. By 42 weeks the efficiency of the placenta is much reduced. All this should be discussed by the individual woman with her own obstetrician so that a decision can be made that is right for her and her fetus.

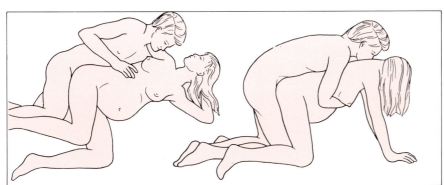

Intercourse in later pregnancy is a problem; the growing lump of the uterus prevents many people enjoying their usual position comfortably. Now, the man may approach the woman from the rear, lying either on the side or in the hands and knees position.

At the antenatal clinic the obstetrician may do the following:
Show the mother that the fetal heart is beating normally *(right)*.

Check at the ankles for retention of water *(centre)*.

Examine the fetus through the mother's stomach wall to check size and position *(far right)*.

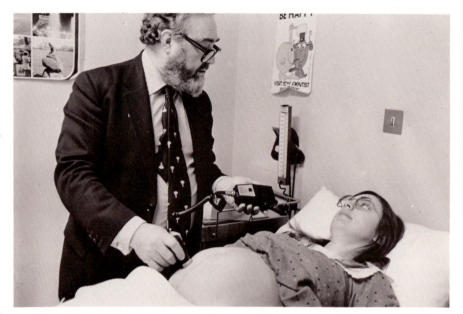

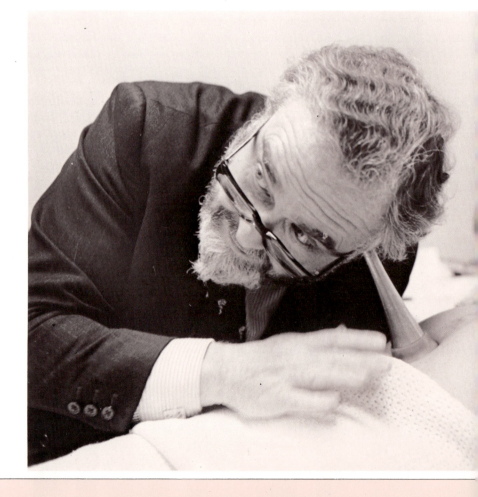

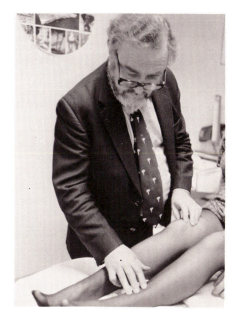

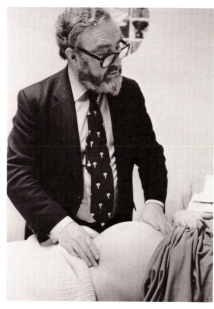

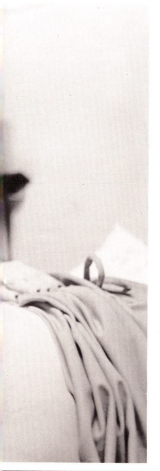

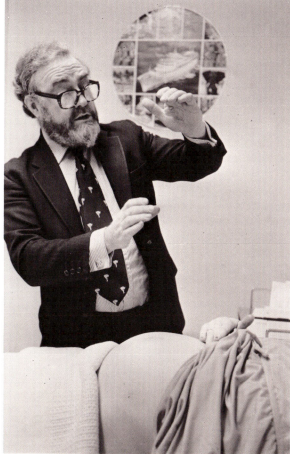

The obstetrician will also listen to the fetal heart with a simple tubular stethoscope (*far left*). (Your husband could do the same with a cardboard tube.)

After making his examination the obstetrician can give the mother some idea of the length of the fetus (*left*).

Multiple pregnancies

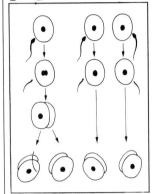

Identical twins come from one sperm, one egg dividing into two (*above left*). Non-identical twins come from two separate eggs and two separate sperm (*above right*).

Twins and triplets are so different from single pregnancies that I have devoted a separate section to them. Instead of dealing with them chronologically as the rest of the book does, all the events raised in multiple pregnancy are grouped together here.

The most common litter size in the human is one baby at each pregnancy; exceptionally two or more may be carried at the same time. The frequency of twins in the UK is about 1 in 100 pregnancies, but it is much commoner in some races: for instance in West Africa the incidence can rise to 1 in 30 pregnancies. Triplets occur 1 in 10,000 births in this country and quadruplets 1 in 150,000. There is much popular concern that the use of fertility drugs which stimulate ovulation artificially have increased the twin and triplet rates. This is not so, for very few women, in fact, are taking such fertility drugs. No exact measure can be made of those using ovulation-stimulating drugs, but probably they are a few thousand only compared with the 600,000 women who give birth each year in England and Wales. Thus, although occasional cases of quins and sextuplets are widely reported in the press after the use of fertility drugs, when viewed in the context of the total population they are rare. If a woman is taking such drugs she is usually monitored very carefully by the hospital supplying them, so that over-stimulation does not often occur.

Types of twin

Twins may be of two types: the first occurs when a single egg is fertilized by a single sperm, and the second when two separate eggs are fertilized by two different sperm. In the former case, the fertilized cell divides into two, a simple division, but this cell mass then divides into two separate groups of cells rather than into a single four-cell stage. Common chromosomal material will be in each of these pairs of cell clumps, so the sex and physical characteristics of babies which result will be the same and so produce identical twins. The twins produced from two eggs are completely separate. The chromosomal material is different from both the egg and sperm so that any babies which result can be of different sexes and physically have no more in common than any other two members of the same family. They just happen to share a uterus at the same time and they will be non-identical twins. They are three times as common as the identical twins produced from one egg.

The differentiation of twins is sometimes important in law. Obviously if

When twins are born, the placentas are carefully examined. If the placentas are well separated (*right*) the twins are obviously non-identical. However, if they are fused together (*centre*), we cannot distinguish identical from non-identical twins, for the two placentas of the latter may fuse together structurally (*far right*).

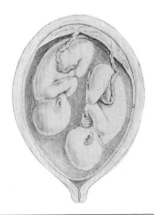
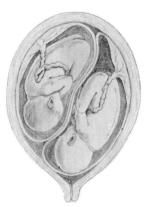
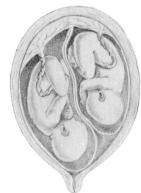

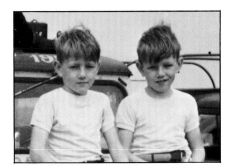

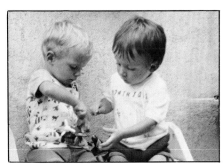

Identical twins (*far left*) share the same genetic material and will be exactly the same. Non-identical twins (*left*) have no more in common than any other brothers and sisters; they just share the same uterus.

they are of different sexes they must come from two eggs. At birth, the placenta and the membranes around it may be examined to see whether the twins share a common placenta or not, but this is by no means absolute. The blood groups can be checked, those of identical twins will be the same for all blood groups. As well as the A and B and O, and the rhesus groups, there are some 15 or 20 specialist blood groups which may be examined in cases like this. Fingerprints are useful, for, if they are different, twins are obviously not identical. However, the points of similiarity are sometimes difficult to see between identical twins. The final test is to check the typing of the antigens produced by the tissues. Each of these is individual to an individual person but if they should be common to two, these two must have exactly the same chromosomal material down to the last gene. This can only occur with identical twinning.

While there may be some suspicion of twins because of past or family history, most twins are not diagnosed until 25 to 30 weeks of pregnancy. Then the examining doctor or midwife finds the uterus to be bigger than expected. Before this time, the uterus need not be obviously larger, for two very small fetuses can share the same space and volume of uterus as one. In these days, more women in the West are having ultrasound estimation performed at about 16 weeks. In most cases, this procedure will diagnose twins or other multiple pregnancies, so that the parents-to-be can be given warning much earlier than was previously possible. After 22 weeks, an X-ray can be taken to confirm twins but this is usually only done if the doctors have genuine doubts and the ultrasound scan is inconclusive.

How will the doctor diagnose twins?

Twins can present in many combinations. The commonest is when they are both head down, next is head and tail, and then bottom and bottom. These three combinations account for 95 percent of all twin presentations. If one twin is in a transverse position difficulties can arise.

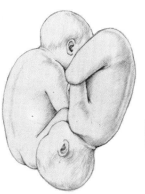

Both head down

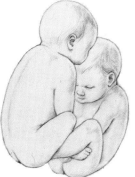

Head and tail

Bottom and bottom

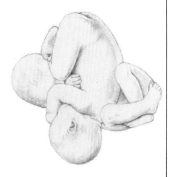

One twin transverse

Will twins make a difference to the pregnancy?

The mother carrying twins will have a heavier load to carry. As well as the extra weight of more than one baby, placenta and surrounding fluid, the body reacts differently to twins than to a singleton pregnancy. The hormone changes are greater in twin pregnancy, causing an exaggeration of response of the mother's physiology. The incidence of anaemia is increased and so extra checks should be made of the blood. Because there is an increase of raised blood pressure problems in pregnancy, the mother with a multiple pregnancy will be advised to rest very much more than one with a singleton. Indeed, many obstetricians suggest she comes into hospital for extra bed rest. Others would consider that the hospital is not necessarily a place where one can easily get extra rest. It is probable that pregnancy will not go to 40 weeks as with the singleton; the average time for onset of labour is about 37 weeks in twins and 34 weeks with triplets.

Giving birth

The delivery of twins may take longer than that of a singleton but it is usually just as successful provided antenatal care has been thorough and the woman is in the care of competent obstetricians and midwives. All twin deliveries should take place in a large obstetric unit, capable of coping with any complication that might arise and where there is a pediatric department in case of problems with the babies.

Twins can lie in a combination of ways but mostly the leading twin is lying longitudinally, presenting by either the head or the buttocks, so that a vaginal delivery can usually be expected. The incidence of operative deliveries is slightly increased, for forceps may be used to guard the head of the second twin, but in most cases a twin delivery can be normal and happy.

With triplets, the problems are greatly increased. The babies are much smaller at delivery and it may be wise to spare them the stress of labour and to deliver them by Caesarian section. This certainly applies when three or more babies occupy the uterus.

Looking after the children

The real difficulties begin once mother and babies go home to the inexorable round of feeds and nappies and washing. As soon as one baby is fed or changed or comforted, another will be demanding the same attentions and the mother will find it difficult to meet all these demands and to find time to look after her own needs. Try to arrange for a relative or friend to help you in the home during the weeks after delivery so that you can concentrate your efforts entirely upon the new babies, and need not be concerned about the general chores of housekeeping and food preparation for the rest of the family.

There is no reason why twins or even triplets should not be breast fed, although this increases the burden that the mother herself has to bear. A

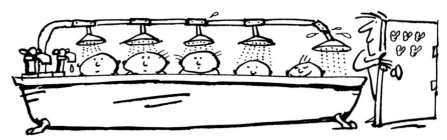

INSURING AGAINST MULTIPLE PREGNANCY

As well as the emotional and physical problems which arise in multiple pregnancy, there are financial ones and many couples decide to insure against these. In the UK, a typical insurance policy would offer cover at the rate of £100 for a premium of £2.50 with a maximum cover of £1000 for a £25 premium. These figures are guidelines only and you should consult a reliable broker to get you the best rate available. A requirement of the policy is often that the premium must be paid more than six months before the birth. Most twin pregnancies do not go to full term (40 weeks) so while in theory the premium could be paid by the 17th week of pregnancy, in more realistic terms the deadline is before the 13th or 8th week of pregnancy.

breast-fed baby can only be fed by one person while the load of feeding bottle-fed babies can be shared with others. Most professionals and mothers believe that breast feeding is the best start for a baby, particularly if he is a little smaller. With proper guidance and support, most mothers can successfully breast feed twins and sometimes triplets.

More practical help can be had from both the NCT and the Twins Clubs Association TCA. Both organizations produce helpful leaflets about various aspects of caring for twins and both may be able to put you in touch with other mothers who can provide advice and support.

The joys and advantages of having twins will, of course, come a little later; you can delight in their similarities and their differences, and in the pleasure of seeing them as the closest possible companions.

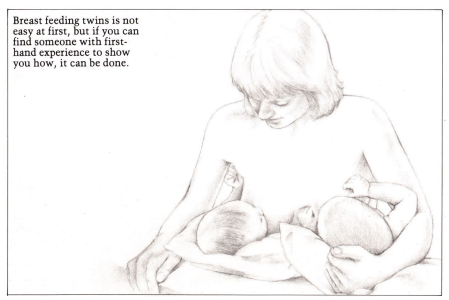

Breast feeding twins is not easy at first, but if you can find someone with first-hand experience to show you how, it can be done.

POSSIBLE PROBLEMS IN LATER PREGNANCY

By the last weeks of pregnancy, all women are feeling the mass in the stomach pulling the body forwards and downwards; tiredness is so common that it is the normal state. In the last two or three weeks, most women are glad to think that pregnancy will soon be over. Along with the pleasure of seeing their new baby will be the relief of not having to carry him around in the uterus for 24 hours a day. Serious conditions in late pregnancy can be greatly reduced if there has been proper and frequent antenatal care. However, there are three conditions that should be considered, even though they are less common these days.

Pre-eclampsia or toxaemia

Pre-eclampsia is a condition of raised blood pressure in pregnancy, a serious feature of which is the passing of protein from the mother's blood through the kidneys into the urine. This is a potentially serious condition that may be life-threatening to the mother or fetus. One of the principal justifications for antenatal visits is the early detection of pre-eclampsia, which can be spotted by blood-pressure readings and the other major check of pregnancy, the early morning specimen of urine tested for protein at each antenatal visit.

If a woman is diagnosed as having early pre-eclampsia she is usually advised to rest. This is sensible treatment: it not only reduces the blood pressure but, also allows a greater proportion of the blood passing around the body to go through the placental bed and so compensates for any reduction, which the pre-eclamptic process itself causes. Should the condition worsen despite simple bed rest, the mother will be asked to come into hospital where other treatments may be given to reduce the blood pressure. In addition, a more intensive watch can be made on the fetus to ensure that he is not at risk by assessing the hormones he is making and by examining his heart rate and its response to external stimuli. The ultimate step in the treatment of pre-eclampsia is delivery of the baby, for the process does not worsen once the baby and placenta are delivered. This cannot be done *too* soon for the child

During labour, the mother rests on her side so that the uterus does not press on the major blood vessels. The fetal heart rate can be monitored by a belt carrying an ultrasound head.

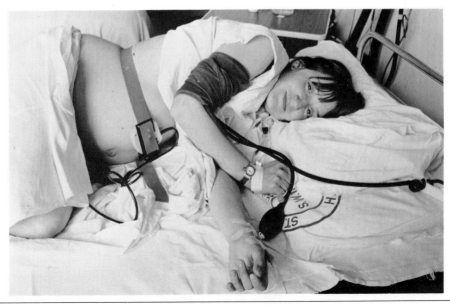

will be immature, but it must be decided when it will be safer for the baby to be outside the uterus, even if less mature than 40 weeks, rather than inside, with the diminishing supply of nutrients and oxygen which pre-eclampsia produces. Pre-eclampsia is probably the most common reason for inducing labour in the West in the 1980s.

Sometimes the process of pre-eclampsia gets worse despite these treatments and the woman herself notices a thumping headache and disturbances of vision. This is accompanied by a sharp rise in blood pressure and the risk of eclampsia, a state of continuous fitting, is severe. In this state the baby is at very great risk and the woman is at severe risk of death. Any headaches or visual disturbances noted by a woman with pre-eclampsia should be reported to her medical or midwifery attendants immediately. In most cases they are not serious and are not due to worsening pre-eclampsia, but this can only be determined by the use of a blood-pressure machine to check that the blood pressure has not really risen.

If pre-eclampsia is dealt with promptly, so that it does not become severe, then the outlook for the mother and child is not greatly worsened. If halted early enough there will be no severe after effects to the mother's kidneys or brain. Severe pre-eclampsia, however, is associated with a greater loss of or damage to babies and mothers.

Bleeding from the vagina

About five per cent of women bleed from the vagina in the last weeks of pregnancy. This is usually not serious but, since some cases may be so, any such vaginal bleeding should be reported to your medical attendants immediately. Do *not* wait for your next antenatal appointment, simply ring your midwife, GP or hospital (depending upon the local arrangements).

Many such bleeds are not serious and come from local causes such as an erosion of the cervix or a varicose vein in the vagina. These can be determined by careful examination at the proper time. The two most serious causes of bleeding in late pregnancy are:

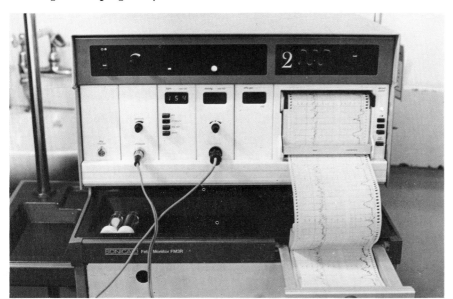

Monitors pick up the fetal heart rate and the strength of your contractions. A miniature portable computer provides a printout and allows midwives to observe how the fetal heart is responding to contractions.

Placenta praevia

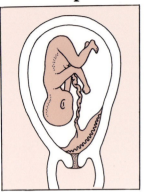

The placenta is covering the mouth of the womb and lying in front of the baby (*above*). When the cervix opens, bleeding would be heavy; delivery must be done by Caesarian section.

This medical term means, literally, a low-lying placenta—here, by chance, implantation of the egg has taken place in the lower third of the uterus so that when the placenta is formed it overlies in the neck of the womb. In late pregnancy, as the lower part of the uterus begins to stretch, the placenta separates slightly from its bed and some bleeding occurs; that blood trickles down and quickly escapes through the neck of the womb into the vagina. The bleeding is usually painless and the quantity small (a teaspoonful or two). It is commonly bright red without any clots and its occurrence should be reported immediately. A small bleed might herald a bigger bleed later on.

The diagnosis of placenta praevia is not made by internal vaginal examination, for such a procedure could cause further separation of the placenta and much heavier bleeding. If the condition is suspected, the woman is usually rested in hospital and, when things have settled down a little, an ultrasound scan is made to show the site of the placenta. Further treatment will depend upon where this is. If it is very low the woman would do well to stay in hospital until the baby becomes mature enough to be born; delivery would then be by Caesarian section. Should labour ensue, a much larger area of the placenta could peel off and the baby would die. There would be much bleeding, probably making the woman exceedingly ill, if not killing her.

The next bleed from the placental bed could be much heavier than the first and, if it occurred when the woman was at home, there might be a dangerous delay in the resuscitation, blood-transfusion and delivery procedures that would be necessary.

In the Western world, with a vigilant group of women reporting symptoms early, the mortality to the fetus and mother of placenta praevia has been greatly reduced. However, diagnosis can only be made if the woman reports the bleeding and this, it must be stressed, is an urgent matter.

Shearing off a normally sited placenta

Rarely, a placenta sited in the upper part of the uterus separates so that a clot forms between maternal and fetal surfaces putting the fetus in danger (*below*).

Sometimes a placenta implanted in the upper part of the uterus separates from its bed. We do not know the reasons for this completely, but when it happens it is a catastrophe for the fetus and can be for the mother also. Commonly, a corner of the placenta peels off and maternal blood floods in to fill the space between the placental bed and the placenta itself. Some of this blood may trickle between the membranes, around the amniotic sac and through the neck of the womb, and appear at the outside world. The blood that appears with this separation of a normally implanted placenta is old, often dark brown or black with a few little clots in it. There is commonly much pain in the uterus at the site of separation and this may be enough to make a woman shocked. As well as the small amount of blood which separates the placenta from its bed, a lot more will have been forced in between the individual fibres of the muscles of the uterus, a painful procedure for the woman. The mother should be taken to hospital urgently. Sadly, the fetus often dies at the time the placenta separates so that, however soon afterwards the woman arrives in hospital, it may be too late to save the baby. In lesser cases of separation, however, the fetus is still alive when the mother is admitted.

A woman with separation of the normally sited placenta will be resuscitated to make her well. If the fetus is still alive and is reasonably mature, a Caesarean section can swiftly remove him from the imperilled environment in which he is now living. Sometimes with lesser degrees of separation, the pregnancy can be allowed to continue for a few weeks but this must be under strict supervision in hospital. The outlook for the mother and baby depends very much upon the degree of separation of the placenta in the first moments after it happens. Since there is sometimes a warning sign of a small separation first, it is for the woman to note any symptoms of this nature — particularly any vaginal bleeding — and report it immediately to medical and midwifery attendants.

Abdominal pain in late pregnancy

In the later weeks of pregnancy women are just as likely to have most of the conditions that cause abdominal pain in, as well as out of, pregnancy. Appendicitis and colic of the gut can occur and should not be forgotten when a woman has such pain. Urinary tract infection is slightly commoner in late pregnancy and this may cause pain in the lower abdomen.

Probably the commonest cause of pain is uterine contractions. All uteruses contract in pregnancy and some women feel their uterine contractions more than others. The differentiation between the painless contraction of pregnancy (Braxton Hicks contraction) and a painful one depends much upon the woman herself rather than a degree of muscular action or even the actual pressure of the contraction measured.

Any abdominal pain in pregnancy should be reported to a doctor. Obviously the speed at which this is done will depend upon the severity of the pain but if it is accompanied by vomiting, bleeding or a leakage of fluid from the vagina, immediate reporting is necessary.

This list of problems may make pregnancy seem like a perilous situation. It is not. Few women get these conditions, but for those who do, the effects can be greatly minimized if they are dealt with sensibly and promptly. Modern treatments, together with the astuteness of women themselves in calling for help at the right time, mean that the vast majority of mothers and babies come through pregnancy happy and well.

CHOOSING A NAME

Most parents find it useful to decide on the name of their child long before he or she is born, or before they know the sex of their baby. Birth can come earlier than you expect, and it is a good idea to have thought about this subject beforehand.

Since you have no idea of the nature or personality of the child it can often be difficult to decide on a name. One simple rule is still important; avoid names where the initials could make up something which would be used to deride the child.

One way to decide is for you and your partner each to compile a list of names without consulting one another. The first name to be common to both lists is the one to choose. Choose one for a boy and another for a girl and then you are ready.

Names go in fashions, but remember that they must last a life-time. Each year the Birth Announcements of *The Times* is scrutinized and last year's most popular names were: Charlotte, Sarah, Victoria, Alexandra, Emily and James, Thomas, Edward, Alexander, Nicholas. Buy one of the popular paper-back books giving lists of names and settle down to read it before making a decision.

GETTING EQUIPPED FOR THE NEW BABY

Try to make your preparations for the new baby in good time. You will probably be too tired to do much shopping in the last couple of weeks and in any case your pregnancy may not go to full term. On these pages you can see most of the items which you will need to consider.

The range of items is bewildering; you may like to draw up your list from a catalogue of baby equipment before you venture into the shops. You may also find good-quality, second-hand equipment advertised in the small ads of your local newspaper.

An armless chair with good back support for breast feeding.

Life can be very boring for a baby — give him something bright to look at.

Draw the blind when you want him to sleep in the hope that he will associate darkness with sleeping.

A changing table like this is ideal for keeping all the essentials together.

An ideal nursery. You will have to spend a lot of time seeing to the baby's needs here, so it is worthwhile spending time planning the room for maximum convenience.

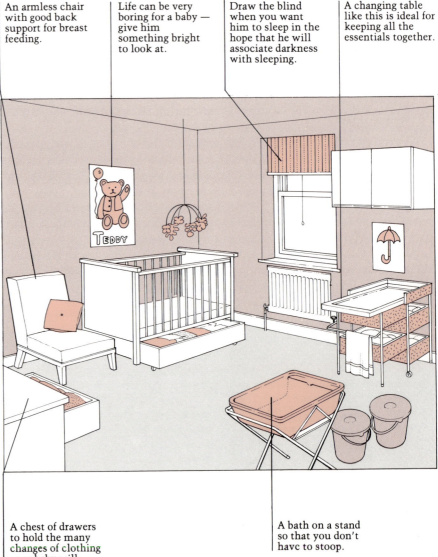

A chest of drawers to hold the many changes of clothing your baby will need.

A bath on a stand so that you don't have to stoop.

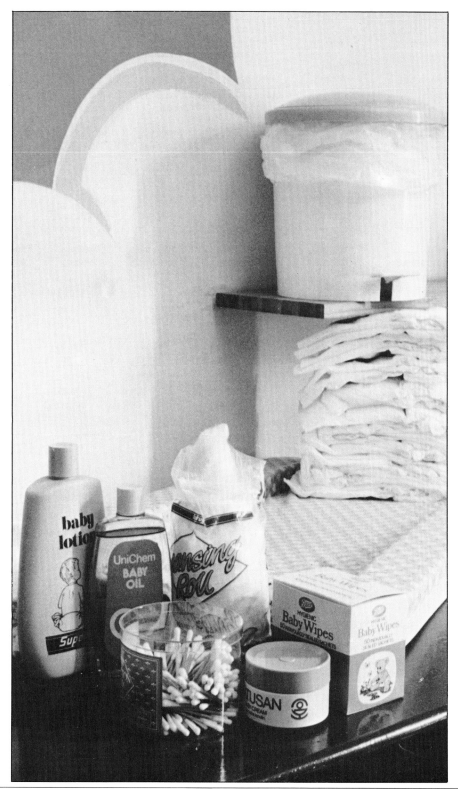

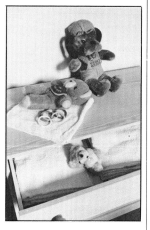

You will need to stock up with some basic essentials for your baby's arrival: plenty of nappies; cotton wool and cotton buds; powders and creams; soft toys of non-toxic materials for him to feel. Although the new-born baby can go straight into a cot, many mothers start off with a carry cot or the top part of a pram detached from its wheels.

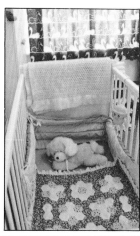

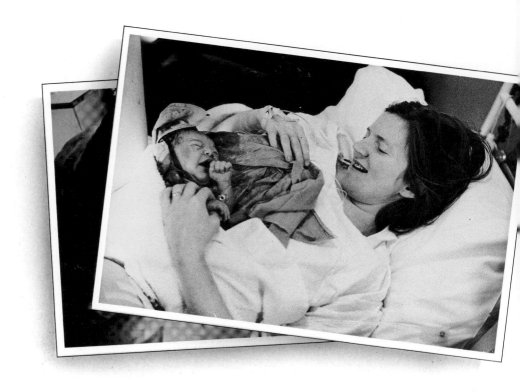

DELIVERY

This is the time that you have been waiting for; pregnancy has passed, some of it happily, some of it rather slowly with the last weeks imposing extra psychological and physical demands. The family is now looking forward to seeing the child and delivery is eagerly anticipated. So eager that every slight abdominal pain is suspected of being the onslaught of labour. This is a normal reaction which no one in obstetrics or midwifery would treat lightly. If you think you might be in labour, contact your midwife or hospital staff for advice. It is far better to ask for help before it is needed than to hang on to the last minute and then have to rush events.

THE ONSET OF LABOUR

It is very important for every pregnant woman to know the sequence of events at the beginning of labour. Labour can start in one of three ways.

Uterine contractions	Uterine contractions become painful over the course of a few hours. In the last weeks of pregnancy, you will have felt some tightenings of the uterus which last for 45 to 60 seconds and then slowly subside. They are not usually painful but may be enough to make you stop walking or carrying on with whatever you are doing at the time. These are toning-up (Braxton-Hicks) contractions

of the uterus getting ready for labour. When labour starts, these contractions become stronger and sharper, helping the neck of the womb to dilate, and pushing the baby down through the pelvis; the combination of these two processes leads to the eventual birth of the child.

Labour contractions are usually first noticed low in the small of the back over the sacral bone and they progress around the side to the front just above the pubic bone. These contractions last approximately 30 to 60 seconds and occur every 20 to 30 minutes. Their regularity and intensity indicate the progress that is being made; from half-hourly, they progress to 20-minute intervals. By the time contractions are coming every 10 minutes, they have a much stronger quality and make you stop your ordinary activities or wake you up if you are asleep at the time.

A show of blood or mucus

The plug of mucus which has guarded the cervical canal throughout pregnancy, or, alternatively, a small amount of blood from the surface of the cervical canal is passed. These two symptoms are caused by a combination of dilatation of the cervix and shortening in the length of the canal. While these commonly occur at or just before labour, they sometimes happen in pregnancy; this is an indication that labour is usually not more than a few days away.

The membranes burst

Throughout pregnancy the fetus lives inside his amniotic sac. In the last weeks, the amount of fluid is reduced but the pressure inside the sac rises because of the increased tone in the muscle of the uterine wall. All that stops the fragile membranes from breaking is their support from the underlying structures. When, in the latter days of pregnancy, the cervix starts to pull up and dilate, there is the beginning of a weaker point at the lower pole of the sac of membranes. When the cervix is fully taken up and starts to dilate, there is an obvious weak point and the membranes bulge through. This provides a much thinner point of the membranes and when pressure rises above a certain point they may rupture.

While labour may start with rupture of the membranes, this is not common. If a woman has never had a baby before, it is unlikely that her cervix will dilate much before labour and therefore the membranes should not be at risk. However, for women having second or subsequent babies, the membranes can undergo stretch after cervical dilatation and in about five per cent of cases labour can start with rupture of the membranes. This can happen

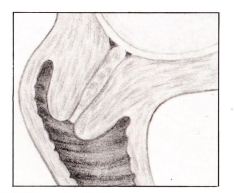
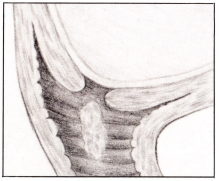

In pregnancy the canal of the cervix is blocked by a plug of mucus which prevents bacteria rising from the vagina. It is usually shed just before labour; you may notice it as a blob of clear mucus.

The amniotic sac, full of fetus and fluid, exerts an even pressure all around the uterus. There is no greater pressure at the lower end than at the sides (*far right*).
Once the cervix starts to pull up, there is an uneven pressure on the bag of membranes in front of the baby's head (*top*). As dilatation continues the pressure becomes uneven (*far right*).

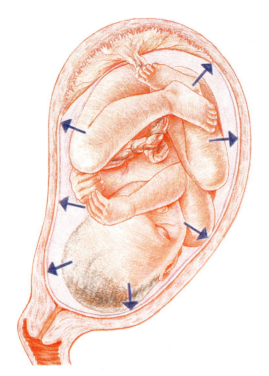

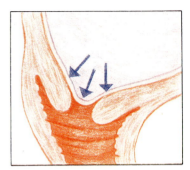

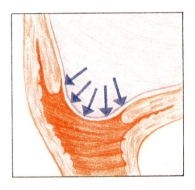

unexpectedly as a gush of warm, clear fluid leaking down the vagina. This is a sign to move to the hospital for labour will probably follow fairly soon. It must be stressed, however, that this is an unusual presentation and very unlikely in those having their first baby.

LABOUR HAS NOW BEGUN

The term labour comes from the latin word *laborare* meaning 'to work'. It is a hard time; the uterus takes the lead and the whole body makes a coordinated effort, lasting several hours, to deliver the baby. Like much other physical effort it is rewarding in its results; you will be tired at the end of labour but happy to have given birth to your child.

Uterine contractions

The contractions come more frequently, building up to about one contraction every two or three minutes. The muscle of the uterus bunches up to help pull on the neck of the womb and expel the baby. You can notice the contractions starting before they become painful but most contractions do hurt at some stage. There is no set number of contractions in labour, but usually someone who has had a baby before will need less effort to deliver her child than one

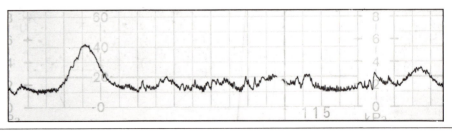

having a baby for the first time. Pain associated with a contraction should not be dismissed lightly. It hurts, but most women take courage from the fact that the pain is a productive one, and is soon forgotten in the delight of those first moments of cradling the baby. A good philosophy is to think of each pain as having come and gone into the past; that pain will never come again and you are now one step further on into the labour.

Conventionally, the professionals divide labour into three stages. They are of completely different lengths and are considered as follows:

Stage 1 Dilatation of the cervix
This starts with the beginning of labour and finishes when the cervix is fully open and is no longer any barrier to the passage of the baby.

Stage 2 Expulsion of the fetus
This starts with full dilatation of the cervix and ends when the baby has been delivered.

Stage 3 Delivery of the placenta
This starts when the baby is born and finishes after complete delivery of the placenta and membranes.

Stage 1
Dilatation

The exact moment of onset of labour is hard to pinpoint. It is when the uterus contracts regularly causing the cervix to dilate. The length of the cervical canal is reduced (effacement of the cervix) by pulling up on the cervix from above. Eventually, instead of a thick collar 2.5 cm long, at full effacement, there is a thin membrane with a small hole in the middle of it. From then on, further uterine muscle effort causes the cervix to be dilated and thus it merges into the wall of the birth canal from the uterus above, to the vagina below.

If a woman has had a baby before, events are not quite so clearly defined as they are for a woman having her first baby; often the taking up of the canal and dilatation will occur together. In some women, a part of the effacement of the cervix takes place in late pregnancy. This can be checked at the antenatal clinic by a vaginal examination; basically, cervical dilatation in late pregnancy is a good thing for it reduces the amount of work to be done in labour itself.

The cervix is dilated by a distension of its circular muscle; it is pulled up by the wall of the uterus above, while at the same time the baby's head pushes down into the opening being made in the bottom of the uterus. Think of someone pressing their big toe against a small hole in a sock; they go on pulling the sock over their foot so that the toe eventually enlarges the hole in the sock and protrudes through the sock itself. With each contraction of the uterus the intact membranes around the baby push further down into the upper cervical canal; eventually they will rupture during labour, if they have not done so before.

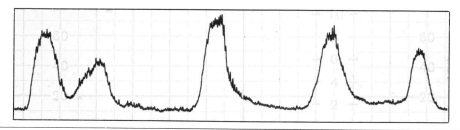

The muscles of the uterus are arranged in a pattern quite different from that elsewhere in the body. When they contract they shorten, as does any other muscle, but as they relax they do not go back to their old length. They bunch up to make the uterus thicker and more efficient at pushing the baby out of his sac. Each contraction of the uterus thus pulls the muscle up a little from the lower to the upper part and so thins the lower part. The uterus thus rides up over the fetus which at the same time is pushed down. The dilatation of the cervix in the first stage of labour and the descent of the fetus do not happen at a uniform pace; dilatation proceeds slowly at first, then gains speed until the cervix is about 8 cm dilated. Another 2 cm dilatation is needed to achieve full opening and this sometimes is a little slower in women having their first baby. Many women feel dispirited in the last hour or so of the first stage of labour and feel they are not getting on as fast as they were previously. This is the natural pace of events and nothing has gone wrong.

Dilatation of the cervix
The cervix is completely undilated and the canal is long (*right*). Towards the end of pregnancy or in early labour, the cervix is pulled up, together with the rest of the uterine wall; a small bag of the amniotic sac comes in front of the baby's head, making a cone which helps to open up the canal (*far right*).

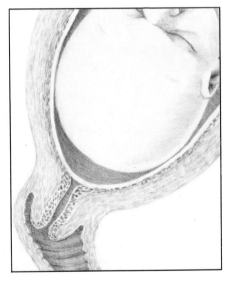 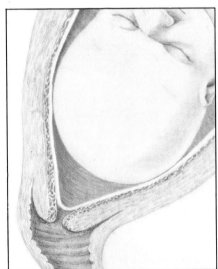

The cervix has started to dilate in front of the cone (*right*). The cervix is now about two-thirds dilated, and both the baby's head and the bag of waters protrude into the vagina (*far right*).

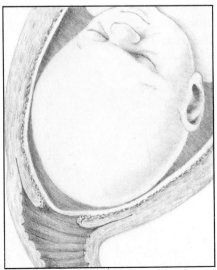 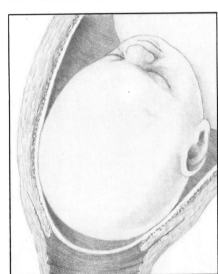

Why do labour contractions hurt?

Pain is something that is appreciated differently by everyone, but for most women, the contractions of the uterus during labour are painful. This is probably due to the extreme tension the muscles generate time and time again with the recurrent contractions. Dilatation of the cervix over the fetal head or body coming down is painful. Finally, in the last part of labour, there is pain as the baby's head stretches the lower part of the vagina.

These unpleasant sensations can be helped by various pain relieving methods (see pages 120 to 123); you yourself may be helped, however, by the simple knowledge of what is causing these pains and what is going to happen in the next few hours. The mother-to-be who is informed about labour usually has a much better time during contractions than a woman who is ignorant and therefore fearful. Fear is a great magnifier of any pain; knowledge can bring calm and with it some control of the pain. By becoming as fully informed as possible about labour, and attending antenatal classes, by discussing fully with your midwife and doctor and accepting modern methods of analgesia, you can diminish the uncomfortable side of labour. No one will pretend that you can abolish pain, but it can be reduced so that it becomes bearable especially when you remember that the end result is a baby, which you have been looking forward to for many months.

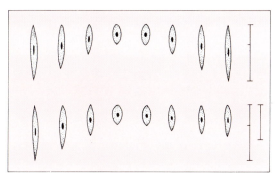
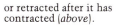

Most muscle fibres of the body contract when stimulated and then relax and return to their old length (*top*). Uterine muscle, however, remains slightly more bunched up or retracted after it has contracted (*above*).

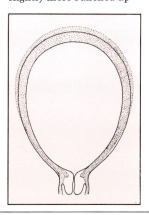

The muscle of the uterus contracts to help open the neck of the womb and expel the fetus. As labour continues, contractions get more frequent and stronger, thus becoming more effective.

The cervix holds the baby in the uterus throughout pregnancy. Now, in a few hours during labour, it has to pull up and open up to allow the baby to pass through (*left*). Your partner's comforting support will help to see you through this time (*right*).

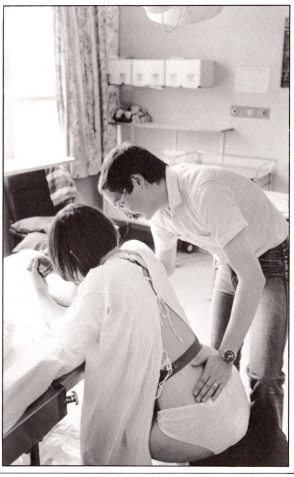

The baby during labour

By the time labour starts, the baby is usually settled into his final position. In 97 per cent of women this position is head downwards. In the remainder, the most common presentation is breech first. The breech may be the lowest part with the legs stretched out to the shoulders or the legs may be tucked up alongside the buttocks so that the baby is sitting in a gnome-like position (see pages 128 to 129).

PRESENTING HEAD FIRST

During labour, the fetus descends through the birth canal and is delivered from the bottom end of the vagina. This journey is not a simple passage but one that involves the fetus negotiating the birth canal, rather like a key turns in the lock in order to open the door. It is best understood by analysing the parts of the descent separately, but remember that in fact the first three take place at the same time, while the last three are in sequence. For a few women these processes start in late pregnancy.

1 Descent The head enters the pelvis with greatest diameter (its longest one) engaging into the maximum diameter of the pelvis (the transverse one). It descends in this fashion to about halfway down the pelvis.

2 Rotation As the head in the middle of the pelvis reaches the muscles of the pelvic floor, the back of the head (the occiput) rotates towards the front of the mother's pelvis, a position designated occipito anterior.

3 Flexion The head of the fetus is pushed against his chest, thus increasing the amount the head is bent forward or flexed. This allows further descent into the birth canal, for the smallest diameters of the baby's head are thus presented to the canal itself. If the head is poorly flexed on the chest, this may lead to a longer labour.

4 Extension As the fetal head gets lower it starts to appear under the pubic arch. By extension of the head as the baby stretches its back, the head is born through the mother's vulva.

5 External rotation So that the maximum diameter of the shoulders can now pass through the same passages as the head, the whole body of the fetus rotates through 90 degrees. This is seen in the outside as a turning of the baby's head towards one or other of his mother's thighs.

6 Delivery of the body The shoulders can now follow, for the head is the hardest and least compressible part of the baby. When the shoulders have been guided through the birth canal, the rest of the baby's body follows easily.

PREPARE FOR LABOUR
Most women are apprehensive when they think about labour, but once it begins there is no time to worry. There is hard work to be done; if you have understood the physical processes involved, you will be well-equipped to work with your body to help deliver your baby. Remember what you have learned about relaxation; concentrate on your breathing, keep it slow and steady to begin with. If you have practised different levels of breathing in antenatal classes, you will soon be able to put them to good use.

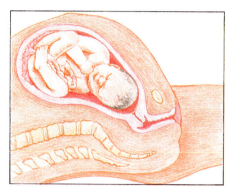
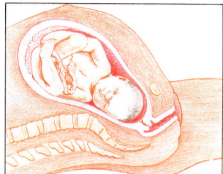

The head descends through the pelvis.

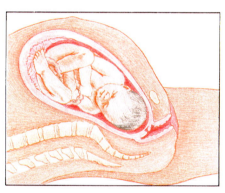
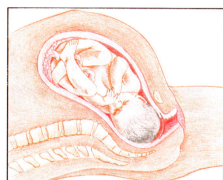

In order to pass through the outlet, the fetal head must rotate through 90 degrees to negotiate the bony passages.

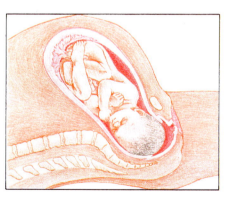
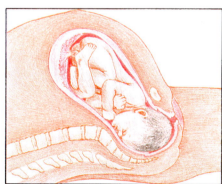

The baby tucks his head against his chest, so as to present the smallest diameter of head towards the outlet.

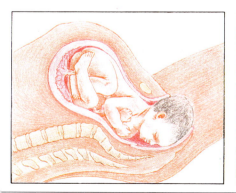
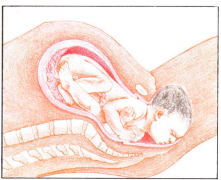

The baby stretches his neck to extend his head as it comes through the outlet.

Once the baby's head is born, the hardest part is through the pelvis; the body follows easily.

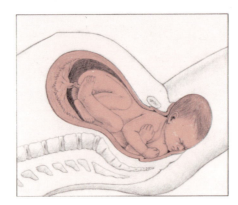
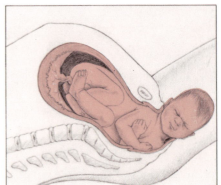
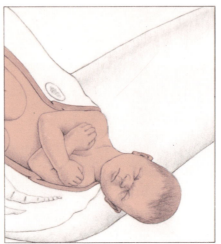
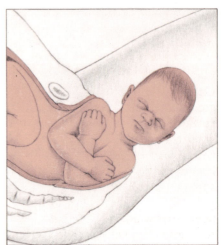

THE EFFECT OF UTERINE CONTRACTIONS

With each contraction, the pressure rises inside the uterus and the fetus is squeezed by the muscle action. This usually has no effect upon the fetus for the pressure is uniformly distributed and he has become used to this during the course of pregnancy by the limbering-up Braxton Hicks contractions (see page 93) which the uterus performs in the last weeks of pregnancy. As well as compression of the baby, however, there is a squeeze on the blood vessels supplying the placental bed. This means that less blood goes to the placenta during contraction, so there is a momentary cut back in the supply of oxygen to the baby during and just after each contraction. Again this is usually no problem and has no'effect on the baby. However, it provides one of the best guides to the baby's well-being during labour, for the midwife or doctor can easily listen to the fetal heart. A special trumpet-shaped stethoscope is used to listen to the heart and this is an excellent way of checking on the baby. The heart cannot be heard during the uterine contraction, but this problem can be overcome these days by using electrical or ultrasound monitoring methods. A fetal heart pick-up may be strapped to the mother's abdomen or a small electrode may be attached to the fetal scalp. Both devices send out impulses which can be transmitted to a cardiotograph — a mini-computer which converts the heart beats into a printout of the heart-rate with a similar

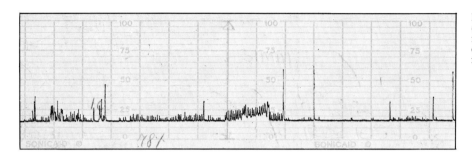

Pressure of the uterine contractions can be measured by a recording device strapped to the mother's stomach.

printout of uterine contractions alongside. The normal fetal heart rate lies between 120 and 160 beats per minute and the responses to uterine contractions usually show a slight variation of the rate. Sometimes the trace warns that the fetal heart is not responding to contractions. This puts the midwives and doctors on alert to watch the progress of the baby carefully.

WHEN TO GO INTO HOSPITAL

Once labour has really started, you are better off in the place where you are going to deliver. For the vast majority this means the local hospital that offers maternity care; for some it may be a GP unit. Obviously, the time it takes to get to the hospital will depend upon the distance you live from it, but journey-time will be affected by traffic and weather conditions. It is, therefore, important not to leave your journey to hospital too late. Many women are apprehensive that they will arrive too soon and that the people in the hospital will think they are foolish for having made the journey at that stage. This is never so, and nobody who works in a hospital ever objects to a woman arriving too early. Far better to arrive early than coming too late and involving everyone in a last-minute rush.

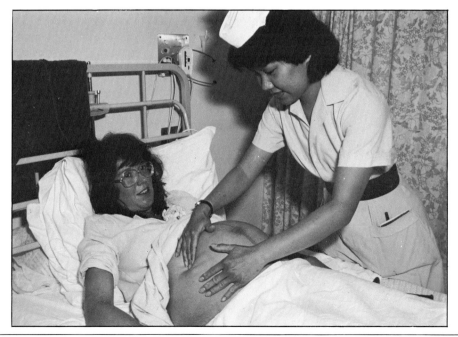

Throughout labour, the midwives will check the descent of the fetus by examining through the mother's stomach wall.

If this is not your first baby the signs of the onset of labour will be more familiar to you and you may think that you are more in control of the situation. However, you must not forget that subsequent babies are often swifter than the first one, so you should not wait too long at home. Of course, you will have other responsibilities, such as preparing meals for the freezer or shirts for the children to go to school, but do not leave the journey to hospital too late; your new baby may suffer if you arrive late and have to do things at a rush.

It is quite natural for you, if this is your first time, to worry about this

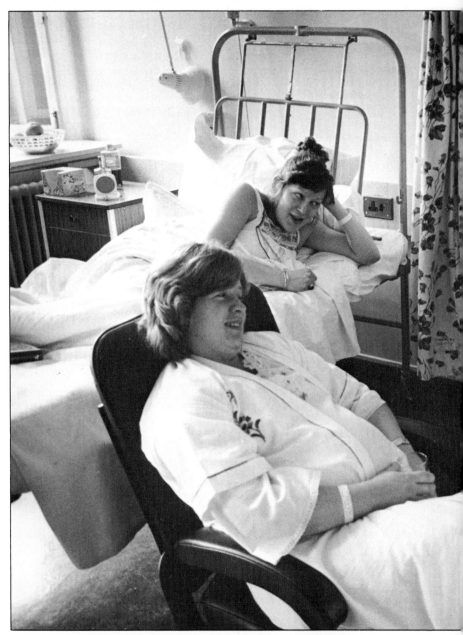

decision. It is probably wise for you to go to the hospital when uterine contractions become regular and are occurring about every 20 minutes. By this time, sensations have usually come around from the back to the front of the abdomen. If the membranes burst and a gush of warm fluid is produced or if there is a bloody show, this is definitely the time to go to the hospital.

For the few who are having their babies at home, the signs that we have discussed so far will warn you to send for the midwife. Again, do remember that the midwife herself has a journey to make and it is a false kindness to leave this too late.

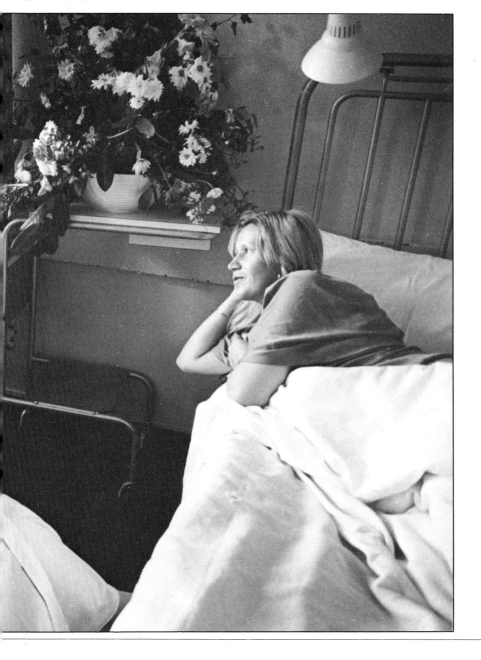

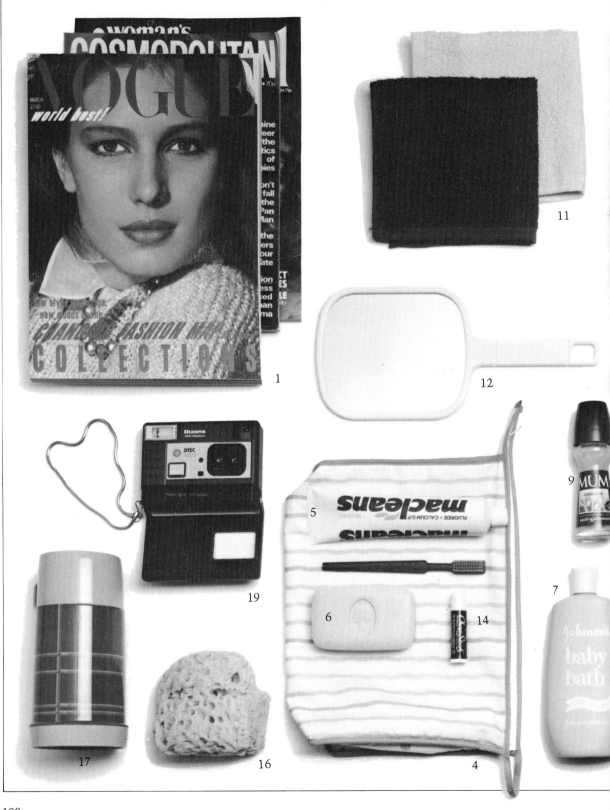

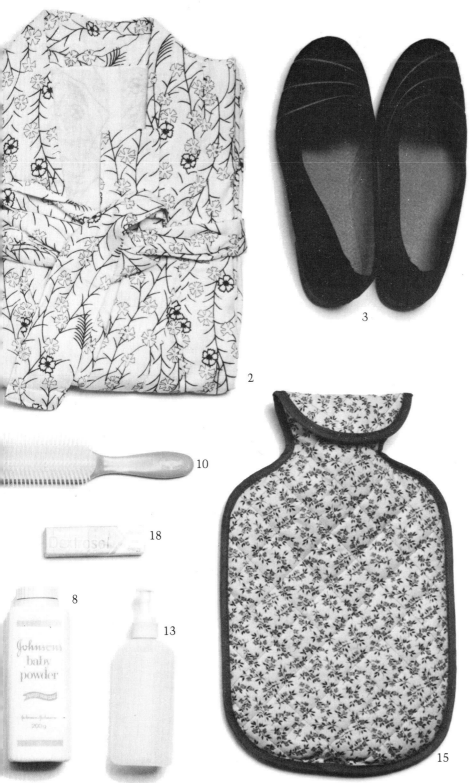

WHAT TO TAKE TO HOSPITAL

If you are having your baby in hospital, about two weeks before your expected delivery date you should pack a suitcase with things that you will need while you are there. These are suggestions for things you will need before and during labour:

1 Magazines and books to read while you are waiting.
2 A dressing gown (hospitals like you to keep well covered).
3 A pair of slippers.
4 A wash bag for your toiletries.
5 Your toothbrush and toothpaste.
6 A bar of your favourite soap.
7 A mild bubble bath.
8 A gentle talcum powder.
9 Your usual deodorant or antiperspirant.
10 Your hairbrush.
11 Two flannels.
12 A good-sized mirror so you can keep an eye on your appearance and watch your baby emerge if you want to.
13 A plant spray filled with water, to keep you cool during labour.
14 Lipsyl, in case your lips become dry or chapped.
15 A hotwater bottle to ease any backache.
16 A sponge for mopping your brow.
17 A thermos flask filled with ice cubes or an ice pack to provide soothing relief.
18 Glucose tablets to give you extra energy during labour.
19 A camera, if you want a visual record of the birth.

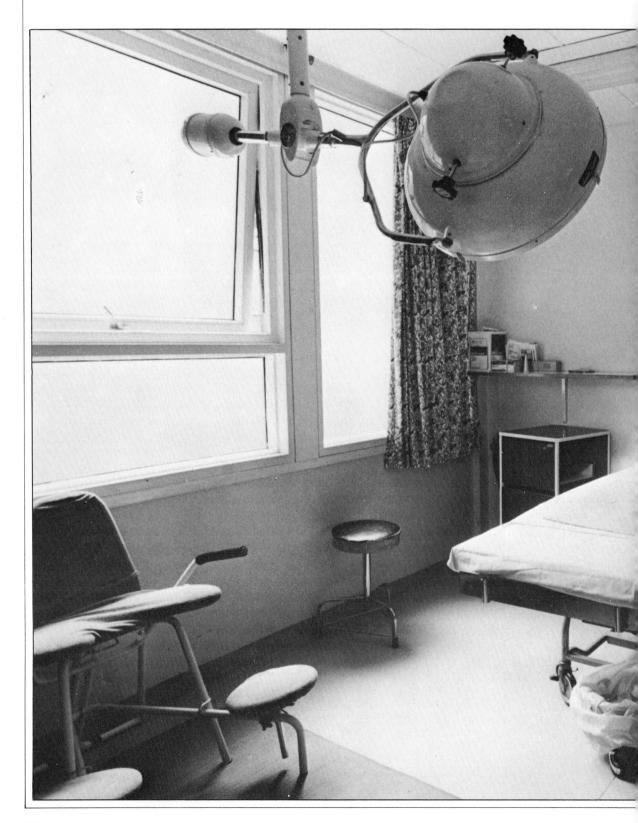

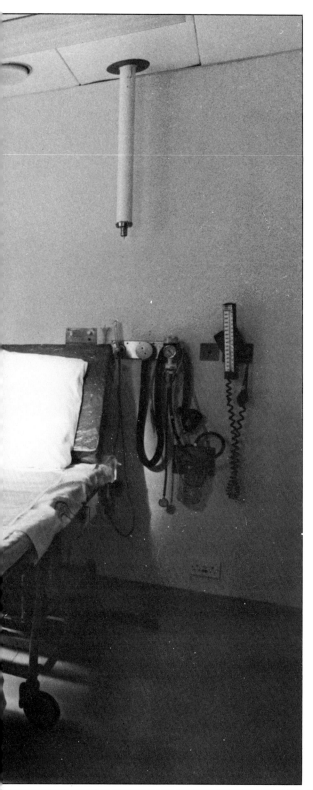

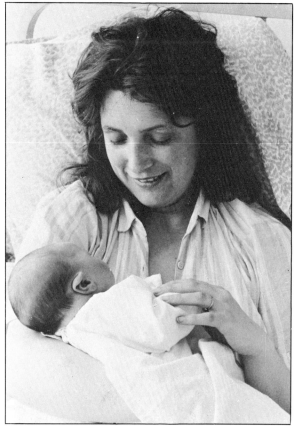

A delivery room (*left*) is a functional space designed to provide all the facilities a woman in labour may need. The bed is covered with a firm, thick rubber mattress and it can be fitted promptly if required. Some women choose to use a birth chair. The big lamp provides the midwife good illumination when required and a pipe set in the wall above the bed head supplies a mixture of nitrous oxide and oxygen if pain relief is felt necessary. It is in this room that the mother will have the first opportunity of seeing and holding her child (*above*).

The support of a partner can be a marvellous boon during contractions *(right* and *opposite)*. While the majority of women deliver on a firm bed, propped up by lots of pillows, some prefer to try other positions such as on a big bean bag on the floor *(centre* and *below)*.

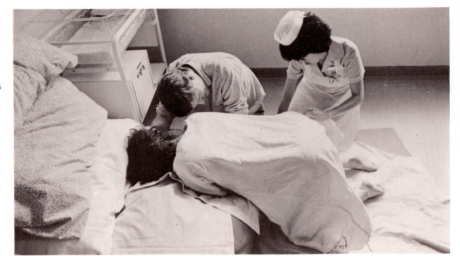

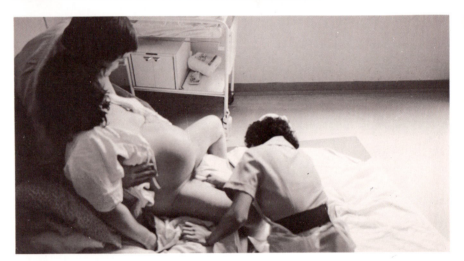

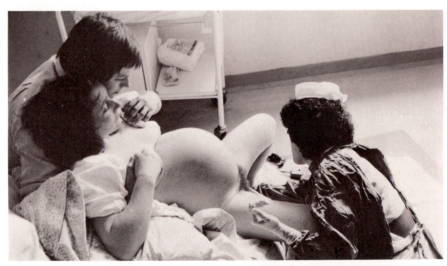

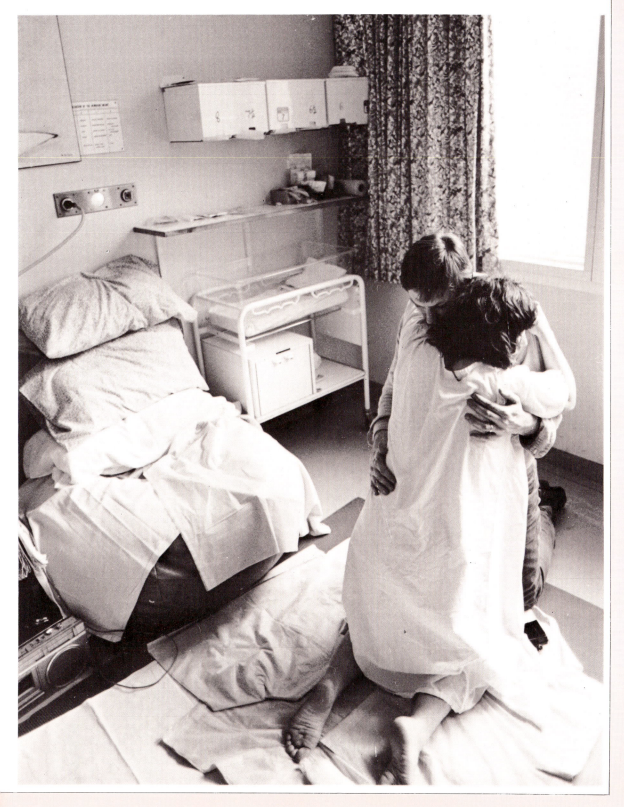

Labour is hard work, after resting between contractions, the husband and wife coordinate pushing. At last, as the baby emerges the father can just see the top of his child's head. Soon the baby is with his mother and father.

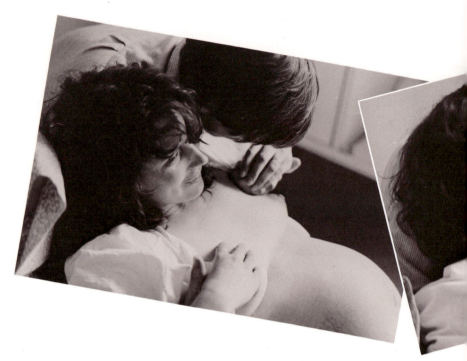

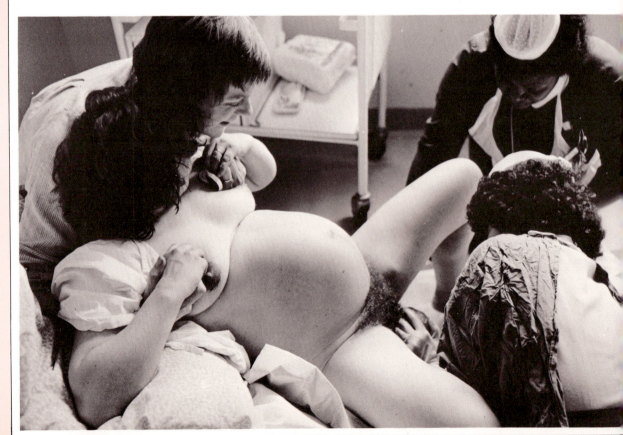

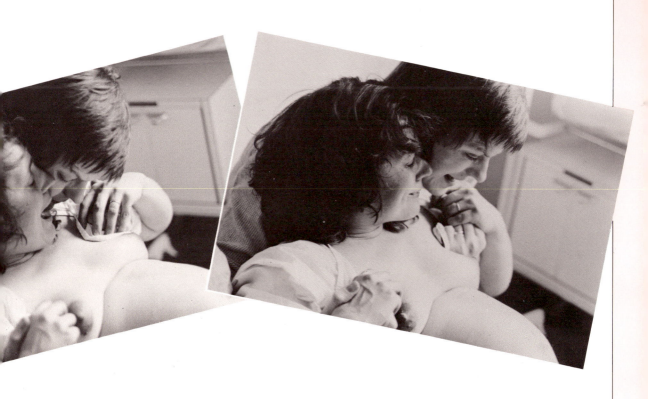

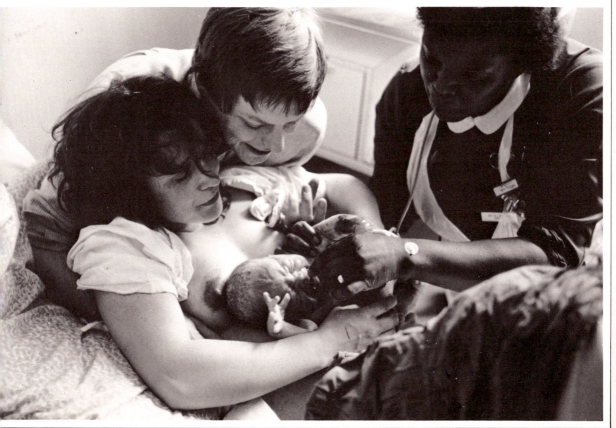

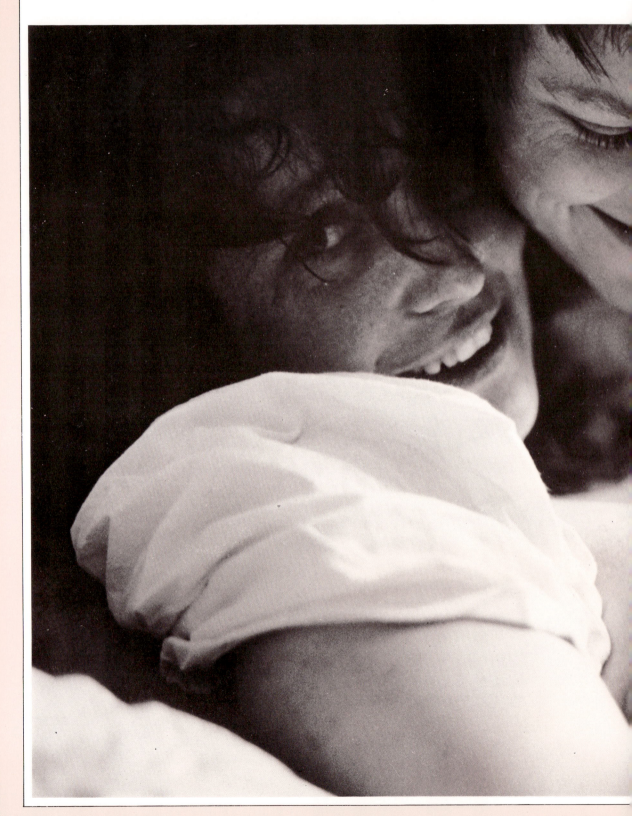

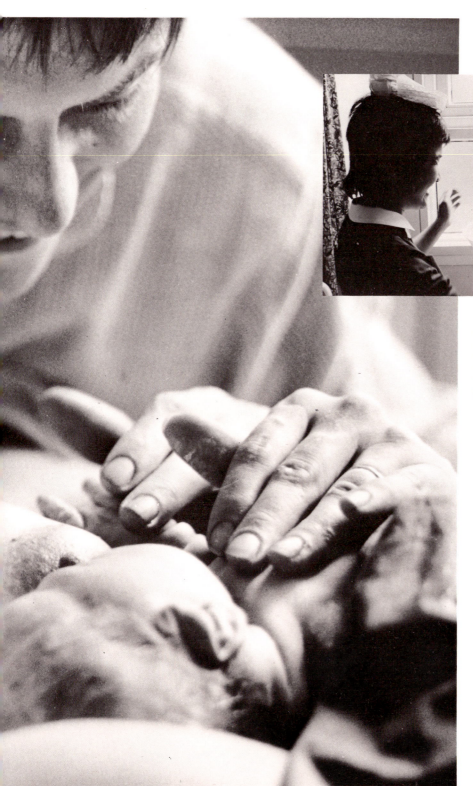

Above: The baby is
weighed soon after arrival.
Birth weight is an
important measure of
nutrition and a guide to the
baby's health in future.
Left: The overwhelming
pleasure of meeting your
baby for the first time.

CARE IN LABOUR

A woman in labour is not treated like any other patient in hospital. She is not ill and therefore is able to do many things that sick people cannot do. There is an infinite variety of patterns of behaviour among women in labour and hospitals, too, differ in the facilities they offer to accommodate this. You should talk to the midwives and doctors who are going to look after you, to find out about the particular arrangements in the maternity unit which you are going to attend, for they may differ from another just a few kilometres away. The pattern considered now is in the middle range, there may be many local variations.

Many women do not want to be confined to bed in the early part of labour. It is not usually harmful for you to walk around so long as the membranes are still an intact sac around the baby. Most hospitals allow you to wander around in the corridors, in the rest rooms, or around your own room in the hospital. You will probably find your partner a great support if he can be with you at this stage. He can provide you with company and diversion while labour is in this early phase.

Later in labour, however, many women want to rest; when the membranes have ruptured most obstetricians suggest that you should rest to reduce the risk of the umbilical cord coming down ahead of the fetus. You do not have to lie down; you can sit in a chair or sit up in your bed. Most doctors and midwives will not want you to life flat during labour; this allows the heavy uterus to press back on the major blood vessels which supply the fetus with oxygen and such pressure might diminish his supplies. Generally, the position you adopt during labour itself will be the one that is the most sensible and instinctive for *you*. At the end of the first stage of labour, however, and in the second stage, most women will probably want to be on a bed.

Most labour wards are equipped with a delivery bed. These are firm, being made of metal with a thin sorbo rubber mattress. They are not the most comfortable places but the delivery bed has to be a practical bed which can be used for the various contingencies that might arise in labour. A sorbo rubber wedge under the pillows keeps the mother at 45 degrees.

Diet and fluids

Some women may feel that with increased activities of their muscles during labour they should eat more. This is not so and it is a mistake for you to eat or drink too much during labour. The usual propulsive mechanisms of the stomach and intestines are greatly diminished so that food and drink are not

---

This is the table of events of a typical mother of 24 having her first baby.

2.30 a.m. Woke up from sleep with slightly painful contractions in the small of the back, coming round to the front, every 20 minutes.

3.30 a.m. Drove to hospital.

4.00 a.m. Arrived at hospital — contractions now every 15 minutes.

5.00 a.m. Internal examination by midwife; cervix opening to 3 cm and contractions becoming painful.

5.15 a.m. Epidural anaesthetic. Pain relief within 20 minutes.

10.00 a.m. Contractions now every 2 minutes and strong.

1.00 p.m. Cervix 8 cm dilated, fetal head well down.

2.30 p.m. Cervix fully dilated, fetal head well down.

3.15 p.m. Normal delivery of male child weighing 3.5 kg.

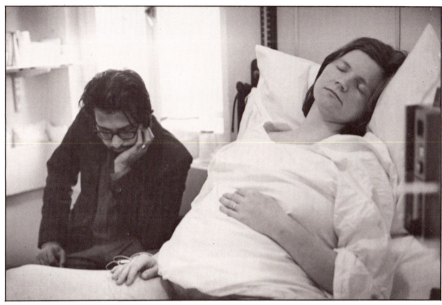

Labour has gone on into the night and the mother-to-be gets some sleep between contractions. It is still a comfort to have her husband there even if he is dozing.

passed from the stomach. Consequently, if you do eat or drink too much, you are quite likely to vomit the undigested food. Most hospitals recommend a light diet and fluid in early labour but later on this is restricted to sips of water. Remember that labour is not going to go on for very long and the reduction in eating and drinking is only for a short time.

Sleep

Obviously the amount of sleep you have in labour depends on the time of day and the strength and frequency of the contractions. If the labour is not very strong and night is approaching, it is sensible to try to get some sleep so that you can wake refreshed and rested when the time for work comes. Lying awake in labour with contractions coming every 20 minutes is not beneficial; sometimes women are offered sedatives in the form of tablets or injections to help a natural sleep.

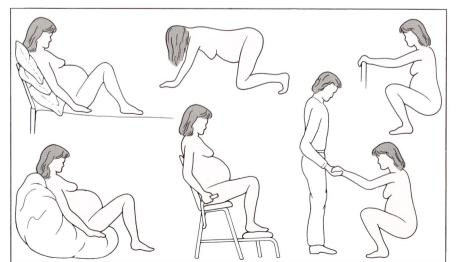

The vast majority of women having babies in this country do so propped up on a bed with pillows or a wedge at an angle of about 45 degrees. A very small number of women choose other positions, such as on the hands and knees, or squatting.

Bowels and bladder

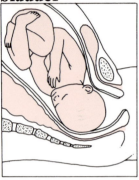

As the baby's head comes down the pelvis, it presses on the bladder and the water pipe in front and on the rectum behind. This may lead to difficulty in passing water or opening the bowels.

In labour the fetal head occupies the pelvis and squeezes the other organs out. The bladder is pushed up and the passage from the bladder to the outside (the urethra) is stretched. This means that some women have difficulty in passing water during labour. If the bladder is getting overfilled it is wise to empty it; if you cannot do it yourself, the midwife may pass a small plastic catheter into the bladder to drain off the urine. This does not hurt although it is an unusual and slightly uncomfortable sensation. By the same token, the rectum may become squeezed by the fetal head coming down through the pelvis; this will give you the sensation that you want to empty your bowel but the rectum itself is often empty. It used to be the practice for all women going into labour to have an enema in the early stages; the idea was to empty the lower bowel to allow a cleaner delivery to follow. The slight stretch of the rectum produced by an enema also had a mildly stimulating effect on the uterine contractions. In most centres this has now been abandoned and most women deliver without an enema. If, however, you happen to be very constipated before delivery, it may be wise to empty the lower bowel with the help of a suppository or even an enema. The best way to avoid this is not to allow yourself to become constipated in the time leading up to the expected time of delivery (see pages 11 to 13 for healthy diet).

Another traditional habit in labour wards used to be the shaving of the woman's genital area before delivery. The reason was to provide a clean area for the delivery of the baby. This is probably unnecessary for a normal vaginal delivery and now most units in the UK only clip the excess hair. If, however, a Caesarian section is required, then the hair on the stomach wall may have to be removed, for there is going to be surgical incision which has to heal. This is undoubtedly better without hair getting in the way.

Pain relief (analgesia)

As we have discussed, uterine contractions can be painful, particularly during the first stage of labour. Consequently, nearly all women use some form of pain relief during this stage. The most commonly used analgesics are discussed in the following pages; you should consider them carefully, discuss the pros and cons with your doctor or midwife and then decide which you would prefer. Once you are in sufficient pain to want an analgesic it may be too difficult to try to work out which would be best for you. On the other hand, you cannot know in advance what the pain will be like and so you cannot make absolute decisions in advance. You may decide early on that you do not want to have any drugs and then find that the pain is greater than you had anticipated. This is nothing to be ashamed of and no one will criticize you for changing your mind. The most common analgesic is an injection of pethidine, a powerful pain-relieving drug which also helps to reduce spasm of the uterine muscles. Injection is usually given in the buttock and it may take 15 or 20 minutes to start working, so do not expect immediate relief. The effect of the injection will last for two or three hours and will make life much more bearable without actually making you unconscious.

The point at which you start using pain relieving drugs will be up to you and your midwife or doctor; no blanket rules can be laid down. You should make your needs known to your midwife, remembering that from the time you ask for pain relief to the time it actually works could be as much as half an hour; you must allow for the getting of the drug, its injection, its absorption and

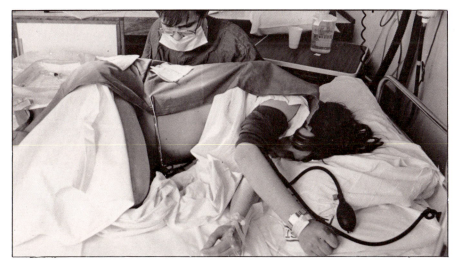

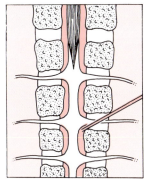

An epidural anaesthetic is injected into the space in the spine from where the nerves flow (*above*).

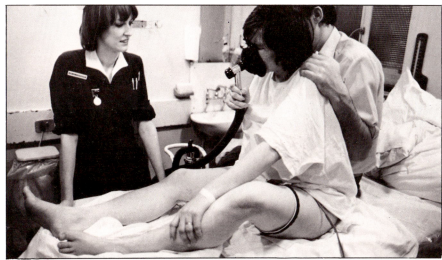

Both nitrous oxide and oxygen are helpful for pain relief in late labour *left*). The woman learns to use the mask before the need is there.

circulation to arrive at the sensation areas of the brain. If pethidine is given too early it can postpone uterine contractions and so prolong labour; conversely, if given late it may affect the start of respiration of the baby after he is born, so your attendants may withhold pethidine at certain times. This is not because they are unkind or being authoritarian, but is in the best interests of you and your baby.

The use of inhalation analgesia is common in the UK, although this is less used in other parts of the world. The most usual mixture is of nitrous oxide (laughing gas) and oxygen. This may come premixed in cylinders, the proportion of gas to oxygen by volume being 50 per cent; thus you are actually taking in more oxygen to help your baby when breathing this mixture than you would when breathing air, which is 21 per cent oxygen. Most women learn the trick of how to use the inhalation anaesthesia mask in the antenatal classes. It has the advantage of acting quickly: after three or four good breaths of nitrous oxide and oxygen you will notice an effect and after eight or nine that effect is quite strong. It has the further advantage of wearing off quickly so

EPIDURAL ANAESTHESIA

Pros	Cons
1 It is the most effective form of pain relief.	**1** An epidural requires a skilled anaesthetist to insert; they are not always available in small obstetric units, GP units or in the home.
2 The woman is completely conscious and has an unclouded mind; she can therefore take part in all aspects of childbirth.	**2** It removes the sensation of pushing and therefore some of the satisfaction a mother may get in the second stage of labour.
3 It has only a minimal effect on the fetus.	

that you can regulate the pain relieving qualities of this drug to the time of the uterine contractions, and be reasonably free between them. Nitrous oxide does not accumulate much in the body but it would not be wise to breathe it for several hours because you would reduce levels of other gases, such as carbon dioxide, which are needed for respiratory regulation.

The best use of nitrous oxide with oxygen is at the end of the first stage of labour. This is a time when the attendants are not happy to give you pethidine because of the possible effects on the baby, and yet the pain of contractions is often at its most intense at this time. Nitrous oxide with oxygen can take the edge off the pain and provide some help for the unborn child.

In the UK the third most common form of pain relief in labour is currently an epidural. This is an injection of local anaesthetic given to numb the nerves after they have left the spinal cord. It is not a spinal anaesthetic, which is an injection into the spinal sac numbing the nerves at their roots in the spinal cord. To receive an epidural the woman lies on her side with her knees bent up well and her head tucked down towards her chest. This helps to open up the spinal bones. The anaesthetist slips the small needle, under local anaesthetic, into the skin and into the gap in the bones to the area outside the spinal sac. Through this needle, he threads a fine soft plastic tube and the needle itself is then removed. All injections are then given through the plastic tube which is usually led up the back and strapped, for convenience, to the shoulder. Local anaesthetic is injected through this plastic tube and starts acting about a quarter of an hour after the first insertion. Each injection lasts for about three to four hours and all can be given through the plastic tube.

Most women who have an epidural anaesthetic ask for one in subsequent pregnancies. It is a very effective method of relieving pain; however, it also removes sensation from the lower part of the body and your capacity to push the baby out will be impaired. If you have an epidural anaesthetic you are more likely to require assistance by way of a forceps or vacuum extraction. There is also a slight chance that your bladder will not work so well for a few hours afterwards and you may require a catheterization on a few occasions. These are lesser problems and the vast majority of women who have had an epidural say they would put up with them for the excellent relief of pain.

An epidural insertion does require a skilled anaesthetist so that, while a 24-hour service of these is available in large maternity units, a smaller hospital will find it very difficult to arrange. You should discuss this problem with your attendants during the antenatal instruction classes to see if epidurals are available around the clock in your delivery unit. Because of the technical skill required to put in an epidural anaesthetic, do remember that

Transition
You may find the period towards the end of the first stage of labour a difficult one. Dilatation is not yet complete, but the desire to push the baby out may be starting. The conflict in this situation may make your irritable and angry with your attendants and with your partner. While not a formal stage of labour, this phase has become known as transition.

from the moment you say that you would like an epidural to the time that you get pain relief can be 40 to 50 minutes. The anaesthetist must come to the room, set up his equipment and put in the epidural; once the local anaesthetic is in, another 15 or 20 minutes may pass before it acts. Do not hang on until the last minute before you ask for pain relief. Try to pace yourself so that the pain relief comes at the time you need it.

Stage 2 Delivery of the baby

Once you have reached the second stage of labour, the neck of the womb is completely open and there is no mechanical obstruction to the baby passing down the vagina and into the outside world. If your attendants are satisfied that the second stage has started, you can now start pushing with the uterine contractions. You will have practised this in the antenatal classes and will know what to do. Generally, this is done best by taking one or two deep breaths in at the beginning of the uterine contraction, tucking your chin down to the chest and pushing down into your bottom. Such a push can usually be made to last 15 to 20 seconds; if the contraction is still going you should then quickly exhale, take in another deep lungful of air and push again. With average contractions, most women can get three or four pushes into each contraction.

Each time you do this, you help the descent of the fetal head down the vagina; with each contraction assisted by your own efforts the head probably advances about a centimetre, but it recedes about a half a centimetre between the contractions, so that the total gain is not as great as it appears. However, each little descent is some progress and pushing with uterine contractions at the second stage of labour is, to most women, a most satisfying way of helping the baby to deliver. Once the baby's head is on the point of delivery, your midwife may ask you to stop pushing so that she can guide the head out in a

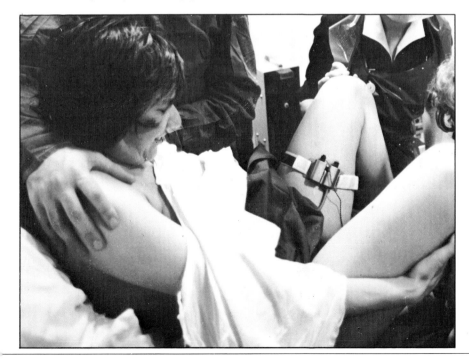

In the pushing stage of labour you can often help the delivery of the baby by pulling up on your thighs with your own hands.

123

controlled fashion. Control is important, for excessive pressure at this time could rush the head through the lower vagina, resulting in a larger tear than is necessary and possibly causing excessive pressure changes inside the baby's head. It is very difficult to be controlled at this stage and the easiest thing to do is to pant. Anyone who is breathing hard with open vocal cords cannot push. This is a trick that can be practised at home and in antenatal classes.

The fetal head descends through the vagina, as described previously, and your midwife will be with you all the time at this stage. When she thinks delivery is getting close, she will wash and scrub up to make sure that her hands are clean, put on sterile rubber gloves and probably a gown as well. In most labour wards the face mask has now been relegated to use for operative deliveries only, so you can watch the expression on the midwife's face as delivery is going on. She will clean up the skin around the vagina with a mild antiseptic solution and put some sterile towels down to accept the baby. When she thinks the baby's head is about ready to be delivered, she may ask you to give a little push, then, very soon after, to stop pushing and pant. It is important to listen to the instructions at this stage in order to help the midwife to help you.

Sometimes, the midwife thinks the baby's head is stretching the tissues and is going to produce a tear of unwarranted size. She may then do an

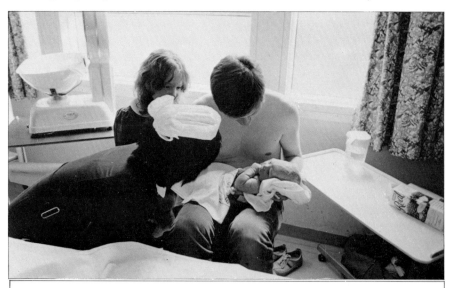

THE NEWBORN CHILD

Babies, like all other human beings, come in different sizes and shapes. The average birth weight in this country is 3.5 kg, but many are much smaller and some bigger. It is unusual for a baby to weigh more than 4.5 kg, but in very rare cases babies have weighed in at nearly 6 kg. They may be long and scrawny or short and fat. The skin will be wrinkled if they are immature, or well padded if mature. Their hair, always a point of great discussion, also varies. The colour bears some relation to that of the parents, but often at birth the baby's hair will look dark because it is wet; after washing and drying it will become fairer and it can change more in the next few weeks after delivery, often becoming lighter still.

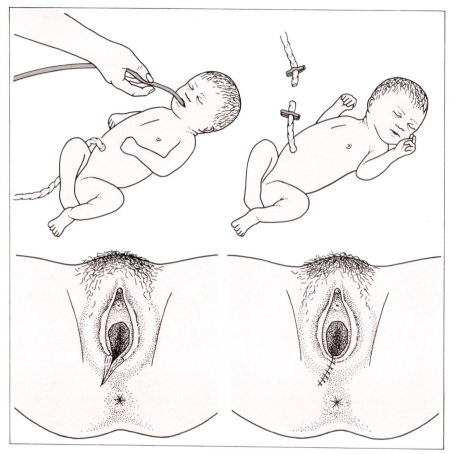

The newborn child has fluid and mucus in the nose and mouth; this is sucked out with a soft plastic catheter before he takes his first breath (*far left*). Occasionally, he coughs up more material after starting breathing; this too needs removal.

The umbilical cord was the essential link between the fetus and the placenta. After birth the placenta is no longer needed, so the cord is clamped and cut (*left*). There are no nerves in the cord so it does not hurt the baby (or the mother).

If an episiotomy has been made in the tissues of the entrance to the vagina, it must be repaired with a few soft catgut stitches under local anaesthetic (*far left* and *left*).

episiotomy — a cut into the perineal skin and muscles at the bottom of the vagina. If an epidural has not been set up, the midwife will probably give a small injection of a local anaesthetic into the skin. Such a cut is usually performed to avoid a tear. In some parts of the world the episiotomy is used on all women routinely; this is not so in most hospitals in the UK — it is used to prevent further damage and stretch of the pelvic muscles. In a very small number of women, an episiotomy is done because the muscles at the bottom of the vagina are actually holding up delivery of the baby. This is less usual but may be considered by your midwife. If an episiotomy or a tear does occur, it will be repaired with absorbable stitches under local anaesthetic when delivery is over. A well repaired episiotomy with properly placed stitches is more satisfactory than a repaired tear.

As the baby is being delivered, the mother is usually given an injection which will help the uterus contract and prevent her bleeding excessively. The baby is now delivered into the outside world, but is still attached to the mother by the umbilical cord. This was the communication link between the fetus and the placenta, the exchange station, which is no longer needed, so it is clamped and cut to prevent loss of blood. There are no nerves in the umbilical cord so it does not hurt either mother or baby. Some people wait until the baby has uttered the first cry before cutting the cord. This is not an essential matter, for circulation to the cord stopped at the time of delivery, the placenta having separated at this point.

At birth the baby's nose and throat are full of fluid. He has been living inside the uterus in a liquid environment so it is quite natural that fluid should still be there. He is about to take his first breath of air so the midwife will usually clear the air passages with a little suction, for it is wiser for him not to inhale any of this fluid into the lungs. Most babies make their first breath within 30 seconds of delivery. They take a deep breath in and then, on the breathing-out phase, often cry, the noise the parents have been looking forward to for months. Soon regular respiration follows and the baby is breathing properly. The few babies who do not start spontaneous respiration quickly will require urgent assistance and this is one of the reasons why it is wise to deliver in a hospital unit. The midwife or doctor may have to give oxygen to the child or even pass a small tube through the mouth to get oxygen in the right place. Less than five per cent of babies require this treatment but, since no one can predict which babies will need it, it is wise to be in a place where the equipment and skills are available.

Once the baby is crying, he is usually wrapped in a warm blanket and given to you so that within seconds of delivery you can be holding your own baby. If you wish to hold the naked baby next to your skin, you may do so, but both you and the baby should be covered with a warm blanket, for the delivery room is a cold place if you have been living in the uterus for nine months. This is a good moment also to suckle the baby. There is no milk in the breast at this stage but it is a good habit to start now.

After hard work, the baby is born. The mother, quite rightly, has the first look at her new baby.

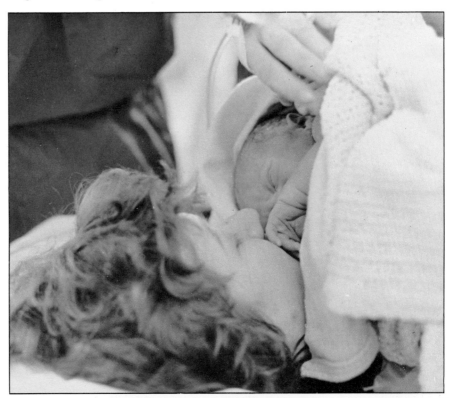

Meanwhile, the third stage of labour has started and the placenta must be delivered. This is usually a fairly easy business after the hard work of delivery of your baby. The midwife will do most of the work and will help you to deliver the soft spongy placenta through the vagina. A few contractions may come at this time and you may notice the uterus firm up as the midwife gently tenses on the umbilical cord to draw the placenta down the vagina. There is usually no pain at this stage. All that remains now is the cleaning up and if there has been a tear or an episiotomy, suturing (stitching).

ROLE OF THE PARTNER

Labour is a time of great stress and one where many women want to have somebody with them whom they know and trust. While there will be professional trust in the medical and midwifery attendants, emotional trust will probably lie with the father of the child at this time. If the father is unable or unwilling to be present many hospitals will allow a close friend to stay with you and support you. In the UK, 90 per cent of deliveries now take place with the woman's husband or partner in the room. If your partner is going to be with you, it is best if he can attend some antenatal classes so that he too is prepared for what is to happen. As well as providing the important emotional support, there are many small physical tasks he can do to ease your pain. He can mop your face and give you sips of water, he can massage your back or just hold your hand and talk to you. It seems fitting that the man who started the pregnancy should play a part in the end result and it is, of course, a bonding

Stage 3 Delivery of the placenta

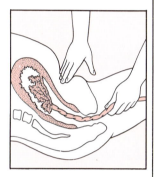

The placenta has separated from the uterine wall; the midwife guides it out, her left hand gently pulling on the umbilical cord, and the right hand guarding the uterus (*above*).

Towards the end of labour, the mother is tired. She is working with the contractions and resting between them. While professional help is important, it is her partner who suppors her most in this stage (*left*). For those who do not wish to be present, labour can be a boring time (*below*).

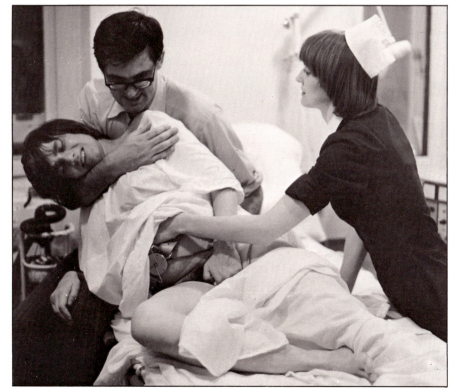

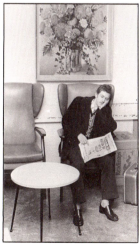

process which many couples feel strengthens their relationship. If you have decided in advance that there are certain things that you do or do not want in labour, your partner will be able to make these wishes clear to the midwife so that you are free to concentrate on what is happening to you.

In some hospitals, your partner may be asked to leave during certain procedures, particularly if an operative delivery is to take place. Practice varies widely from one hospital to another, so discuss this in the antenatal period with the midwives and doctors who will be looking after you.

PROBLEMS IN LABOUR

Four out of five women who have a baby in this country do so quite normally and run into no problems in labour. They labour at about the right time, have about 8 to 12 hours of contractions and then, with a little assistance from a midwife, have a normal delivery of a normal baby. Among the others, however, problems may arise.

Delay in labour

Some women start labour with no problems but then find that the contractions of the uterus are too weak or too infrequent. These conditions often go together and consequently there is not enough uterine effort to help the cervix to dilate and the baby to be delivered. This can be helped by stimulation of the uterus. A substance like the natural hormone produced by a woman's own pituitary gland is inserted into a vein with a small needle. This stimulates contractions and often such a woman will go on to vaginal delivery although she may require assistance at the actual point of delivery.

Less commonly in this country, delay in labour is due to an obstruction of the baby's head passing through the woman's pelvis. This used to be a common problem but it is now usually ruled out by good antenatal care. If the baby's head does not engage in the last weeks of pregnancy, or if the doctor's internal examination indicates some diminution in the woman's bony pelvis, action is taken before labour starts to ensure that the baby and mother will not be harmed by delivery. In an extreme case, this will mean a Caesarean section before labour starts, so that the baby does not even try the pelvis. In borderline cases, the doctor may consider that with uterine contractions the head may flex better and thus pass through the pelvis. In consequence, a trial of labour may be performed; this must be done in a properly equipped obstetrical unit where an obstetrician is always available; if the trial does not work, the baby can always be delivered by Caesarean section after the woman has tried for a few hours.

Paradoxically, a delay in labour can occur if the uterine contractions are too strong but are not coordinated and not useful in helping the cervix to dilate. Such very strong contractions can be eased by epidural analgesia but, if that does not work, the fetus will not stand many hours of such contractions and neither will the woman. Consequently a Caesarean section may be required.

MALPRESENTATIONS

Breech

While the vast majority of babies present by the head, about three per cent of them come buttocks first. The breech presentation is more difficult but, provided proper precautions have been taken in the antenatal period, and the woman is in the hands of a competent obstetrical team, there is no reason for any more complications. Labour is often a little longer, and there is more manoeuvring to be done at the end, but the obstetrician will deal with this. The baby comes down with the buttocks first and these are not such an efficient dilator of the cervix. If a baby is sitting with the knees flexed, the feet will come alongside the buttocks and are delivered first. The doctor then helps out the buttocks and the back of the child which usually rotates to allow the shoulders to be delivered. The head, the hardest and last part to come, is the most difficult and this is usually eased out with a pair of obstetrical forceps. Unless there is an epidural anaesthetic the doctor usually gives a pain-relieving injection to the nerves around the pelvis just before delivery and a healthy baby is born. The delivery of the placenta is the same as for a head delivery. An episiotomy is usually needed with a breech delivery and this, of course, must be repaired as already described.

Transverse lie

These are rare; the baby instead of lying longitudinally, lies across the uterus. It is impossible to deliver such a child vaginally and the doctor will usually do a Caesarian section to help this child out.

Occipito-posterior positions

It sometimes happens that the baby's head rotates not as described previously with the back of the head (occiput) going towards the front of the pelvis but going backwards. This is a variation of normal behaviour. It does mean that labour will probably be longer and therefore the obstetrician may advise the use of an epidural anaesthetic. Most babies in occiput-posterior positions deliver vaginally with a little help from the obstetrician and the babies are usually no worse off than the occipito-anterior children.

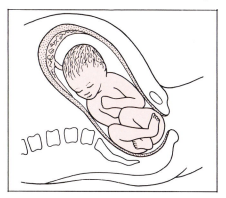 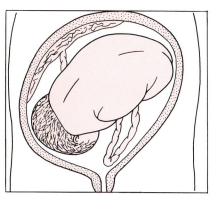

Sometimes the baby does not present head first. When he is presented as a breech (*left*), the buttocks appear first with the legs tucked up against his abdomen. If labour occurred while he was lying almost transversely (*right*), he could not be born vaginally.

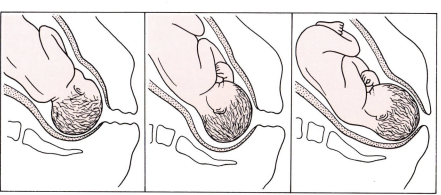

Instead of the head rotating to the front (occipito-anterior) it is rotated against the mother's sacrum (occipito-posterior). This is a more difficult position for delivery.

Face presentations

Rarely, instead of the top of the baby's head coming first (*right*), the neck is fully extended so that the face is coming down (*far right*). A delivery is usually still possible, but if the chin is facing the mother's spine it is difficult.

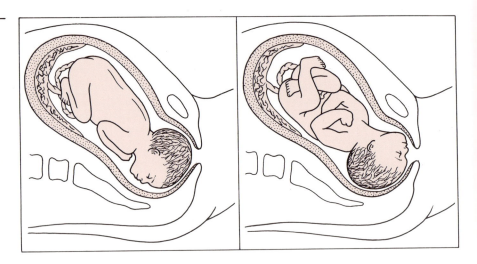

This is another rare presentation where the head instead of flexing as we have described, extends so that the baby appears to be looking straight downwards. Delivery of face presentation is usually normal but it can lead to some problems and may require assistance with forceps.

FETAL DISTRESS

While the unborn child is in good state the fetal heart rate is found to be within a normal range. If some of the methods described on pages 104 to 105 are used to record the fetal heart continuously, they can show how the fetus is responding to the uterine contractions. If there are changes in the fetal heart rate this may indicate that the baby is becoming short of oxygen. Such a condition may arise after a pregnancy complicated by pre-eclampsia when the exchange of oxygen from the placenta is less efficient. Alternatively, it may be that labour has gone on too long for that individual fetus and he is beginning to show signs of oxygen deficiency.

The early stages of fetal distress are not dramatic and the baby is quite safe at the moment; however, he is showing signs of not wishing to stay in the uterus much longer. The doctors may do further tests by checking a small sample of blood from the fetus or they may act on the fetal heart rate alone. If they think that the danger is so great that the fetus will not stand the remaining minutes or hours of labour, they will recommend a Caesarian section to remove the fetus from the low-oxygen atmosphere. In most obstetrics units this can be performed within a matter of minutes, so in most instances the baby is not affected by fetal distress.

MATERNAL DISTRESS

This is a rare condition in this decade, but it used to arise when labours went on for hours or even days, leaving the woman tired out, dehydrated and exhausted. Today it is very rare for labour to go on for that long; most women are looked after well and midwives do not allow them to get to this state. Part of this distress used to come from women's own anxiety and dread of labour. The treatment of maternal distress was usually support to help the mother overcome her dread and fear, the use of proper pain relief and support for the rest of the labour; in extreme cases a Caesarean section was required. If you have taken the trouble to go to antenatal instruction classes and have discussed labour fully with your midwife this is very unlikely to happen.

PROBLEM DELIVERIES

The vast majority of women will have a normal delivery. However, a few will require assistance by obstetricians trained to help when needed.

Occasionally, a fetus will be endangered by staying in the uterus. This may be because placental transfer of oxygen and nutrients have been reduced by some pathological process like pre-eclampsia or a bleed behind the placenta. Sometimes, the pregnancy goes on for longer than nature intended and the baby is again put at risk by staying more than two weeks beyond the properly calculated delivery date. It is for this reason that it is important to get the dates right at the beginning. Any mistake early on could lead doctors to believe that you have reached full term when, in fact, you have another week or two to go. In a few cases, it is considered wise for the baby to come out well before the due date, for example in diabetes where the size of the baby adds to the problems, or in rhesus problem where the antibodies passing across the placenta will increase in the last weeks of pregnancy. For any one of these reasons, the obstetrician may consider that it is safer for the fetus to be outside the uterus, under the care of pediatricians, rather than inside the uterus with the increasing hazard, whatever that may be. An induction of labour may be suggested and the woman can discuss this with her doctor. If induction is to take place, the woman usually comes in to her hospital and one of several methods is used.

1 Breaking the waters A gentle vaginal examination is performed and a fine plastic rod is passed up through the cervix to snag the membranes around the baby. This allows a loss of fluid and labour usually starts a few hours later.

2 Infusion of uterine-stimulating hormone A small needle is passed into a vein and syntocinon, a hormone similar to the natural oxytocin made by the woman's pituitary, is infused. Again after a few hours she usually starts contracting. Sometimes this method is combined with that of snagging the membranes.

3 Prostaglandin pessaries A small pessary, about a centimetre in length, is passed into the vagina at a gentle vaginal examination. Such pessaries contain a hormone similar to that produced by the cervix once labour starts and so help the cervix to ripen and the uterus to contract.

Once labour starts, there is little difference between an induced labour and a spontaneous one. The contractions are not more painful, nor are they stronger. They are the same as spontaneous labour. However, since the doctor felt there was a need to start labour, there are obviously some high-risk features present, so continuous monitoring of the baby's heart may be necessary and a forceps delivery becomes more likely. This is not because of the induction, it is because of the condition which prompted the induction.

Induction of labour

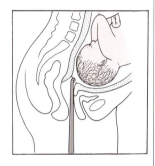

If the cervix is dilated enough, the membranes may be snagged with a small plastic hook allowing the waters around the baby to drain away and so speed up uterine contractions.

Forceps delivery

Occasionally in the second stage of labour, once the cervix is fully dilated, the obstetrician thinks the baby should be delivered faster than nature and the woman are working. The most common reason for this is fetal distress. The baby's delivery is then accelerated so that the shortage of oxygen will not affect him. A pair of carefully constructed guides are placed on either side of the baby's head and the baby is eased from the vagina. Forceps look formidable when seen out of context. They are, however, well designed instruments that have been used for over 300 years in the Western world and they have saved millions of babies from death or spastic conditions due to lack of oxygen. Only the hollowed out end enters the woman; the rest, the handles, are outside and are used by the obstetrician to position the baby for delivery. Forceps delivery takes place with some form of anaesthetic to the nerves of the pelvis and most women experience no more pain at a forceps delivery than they do in a normal one. The blades slip easily into position and have a limited closing action, thus protecting the baby's head and not squeezing it.

A pair of forceps (*example far right*) is a curved guarded instrument the blades of which fit on either side of the fetal head (*right*). The obstetrician can then apply a gentle traction to deliver the baby.

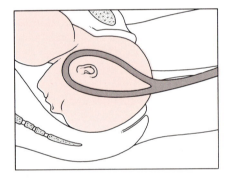
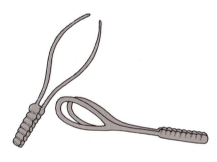

Vacuum extraction

In some centres, delivery is precipitated by the use of a vacuum extractor if the fetus is not progressing at the normal rate. A metal cap is placed over the baby's scalp and air is evacuated from it by a vacuum pump. The soft skin of the head fills the space and provides a button on which the obstetrician puts some traction; this allows the baby's head to rotate and follow the normal line down the pelvis to be delivered. None of the tissues inside the skull — the brain — is affected in this process; after delivery by vacuum extraction there is a small raised area on the baby's head which fades, usually within 48 hours.

A cap from which the air has been evacuated fits onto the baby's head (*right*). The obstetrician pulls gently to deliver the baby. The baby will have a raised patch on his scalp for about 24 hours after delivery (*far right*).

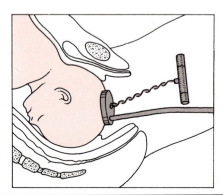
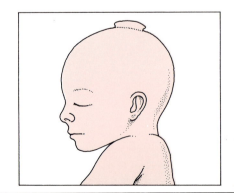

Caesarean section

In the UK, one in ten women are now delivered by Caesarean section. This may be done as a planned procedure before labour (elective Caesarean) or as an emergency once labour has started. The most common reason for the former are conditions which, in the opinion of the obstetrician, would put the baby in danger were he subjected to uterine contractions; these include severe disproportion of size between the baby and the mother's pelvis, a placenta praevia or a previous history of babies having been in severe danger or even dying in early labour. An emergency decision for a Caesarean section might be as a result of fetal distress in the first stage of labour. At this point the cervix is not fully dilated and so a vaginal delivery cannot yet take place.

Under anaesthesia an incision is made low in the stomach and the baby is delivered from the uterus. The anaesthetic may be either full, or, if you wish and there is time, epidural. The epidural anaesthetic allows you to be awake, and in many hospitals your partner can be with you and you will both be able to hold your baby as soon as he is born, just as you would with a vaginal delivery.

There is some discomfort in the days after delivery for there has been an operation with an incision on the stomach but, since the mother is usually fit and well, she recovers quicker from a Caesarean section than from other abdominal operations and, with good midwifery care, there is no reason why breast feeding should be postponed.

These procedures are not normal; they are only carried out when there is a strong need for them. Most women take the attitude that what they want is a normal baby rather than a normal delivery. For most, the essential thing is to leave hospital a few days after delivery with a healthy child in their arms and they trust their doctors and midwives to advise them as to the best way of delivering their child in their individual circumstances.

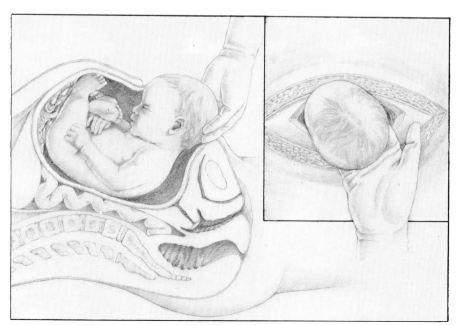

At a Caesarian section an opening is made in the mother's stomach wall and uterus. The baby is then helped out of the uterus head first.

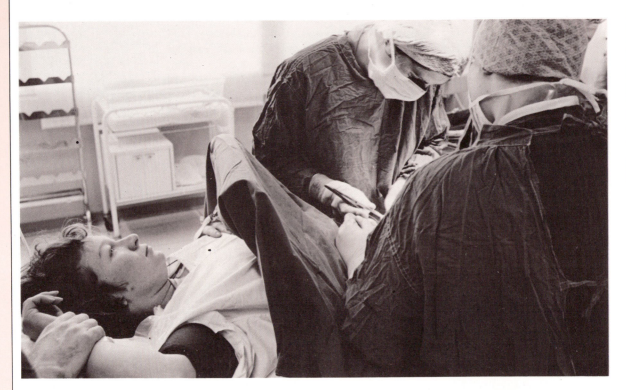

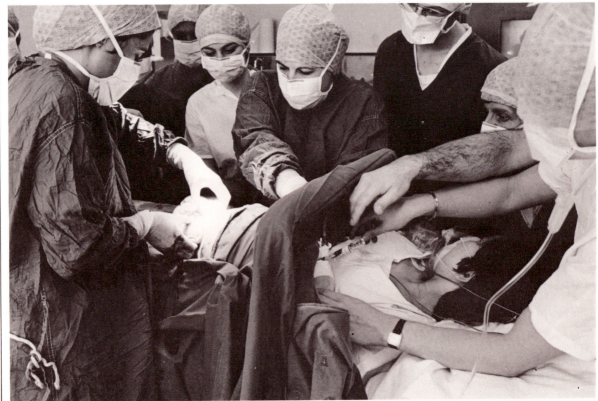

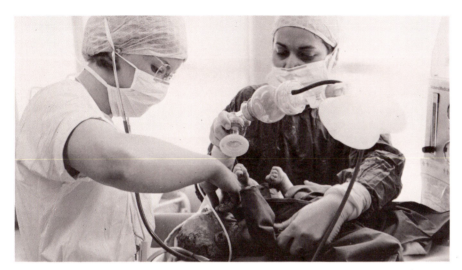

A Caesarean section under epidural
While the obstetrician is operating the mother is wide awake below the screen *(opposite above)*. The baby is delivered *(opposite below)* and after a few puffs of oxygen *(left)* is given to the mother *(centre)* while the surgeons continue sewing up. The baby goes to the breast *(bottom left)* as the surgeons finish and the relieved father lets the family know all is well *(below)*.

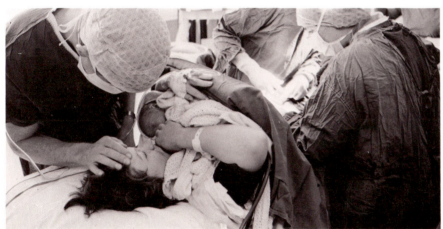

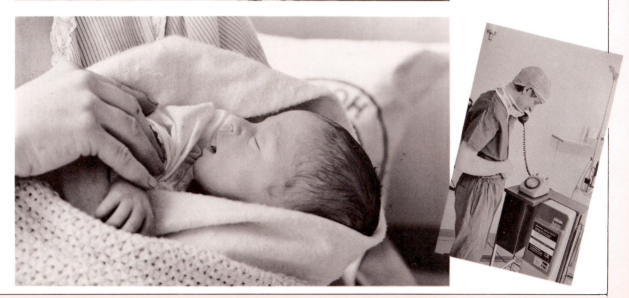

What if labour comes too soon?

The vast majority of women deliver mature babies after 36 weeks of pregnancy. A small number (1 in 25) deliver before this time. Obviously, the earlier the child leaves the uterus the less mature he will be and so the more problems may arise. Pre-term labour is one of the major threats to the newborn in the UK. In most cases the cause is not known, although a spontaneous, too early, rupture of the membranes is associated with some, while inefficiency of the cervix is associated with others. In a small number the doctor starts labour very early because of the risks to the baby, for example in rhesus disease or pre-eclampsia. Twins commonly start earlier and so should be considered in this group.

The management of a pre-term labour depends very much upon where it is taking place and so upon the facilities available to the doctors. The stage in pregnancy in which it has happened is also important. If a woman is in established pre-term labour at 32 weeks in a hospital that has a good neonatal unit, she will probably be able to continue the labour and deliver a small but perfect baby who will be looked after well. That baby may have to go to a Special Care Baby Unit in the same hospital and will have an excellent chance of survival. However, should the same woman deliver in a small, isolated GP

Low birth weight infants (under 2.5 kg) require extra help. They are usually kept in an incubator to keep them warm, to provide them with oxygen and to reduce infection. Various electronic devices are used to monitor heart beat and respiration. They may require tube feeding for they cannot swallow easily.

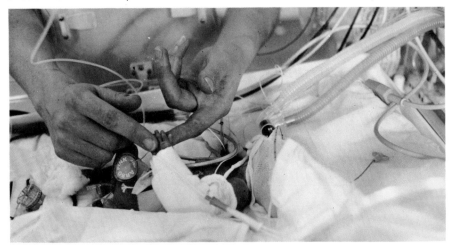

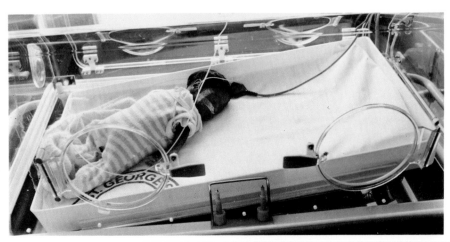

unit or, worse, in the home, then the chances for that baby are very much reduced. If labour is much before this time, the doctors will probably try to stop contractions by giving blocking substances which reduce the excitability of the uterus. These sometimes work, giving the fetus a couple of weeks longer before birth, greatly improving the baby's chances. Further, such a postponement will allow the mother to move from a less appropriate place of delivery to a centre where they have a proper neonatal pediatric unit.

Any woman who considers herself to be in labour should always take advice from her midwife, however early in pregnancy it may be. The sensation of warm fluid flowing down the vagina; or of uterine contractions coming regularly — such symptoms should be taken seriously and not put to one side. The professionals are there to help you and advise you. It may well be that what is happening is not serious and you are not really in labour, but such a diagnosis is best made by the professionals rather than by yourself.

The end results for premature babies bear a strong relationship to their maturity. In the last 20 years, the obstetricians and pediatricians have made great advances and now 50 per cent of the babies born at 28 weeks are surviving in properly equipped and intensively staffed units. They will do so

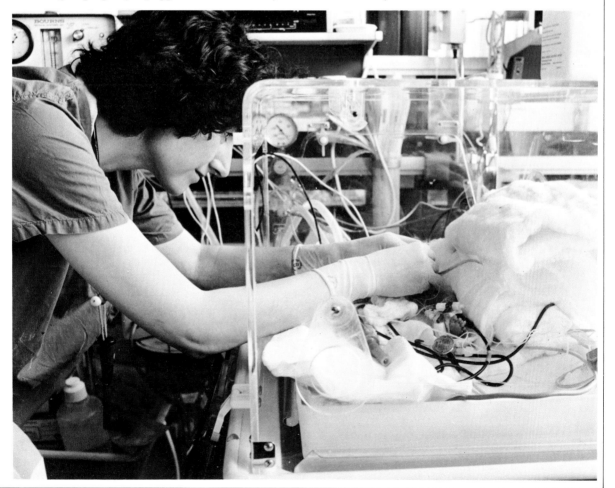

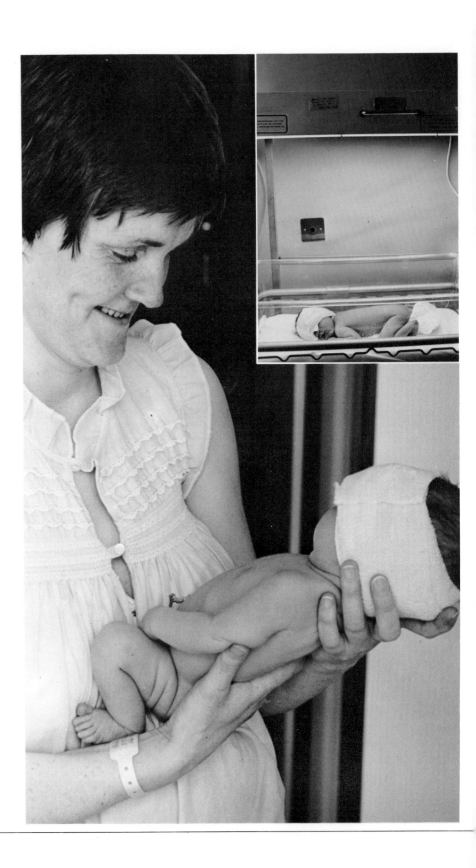

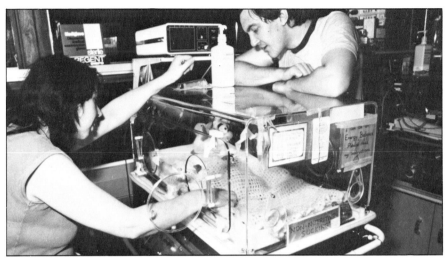

The premature baby is not only smaller than the mature one, he looks entirely different. He is scrawnier and appears under-nourished because less fat has been laid down.

because of the dedication and care of the nursing staff and doctors who work there. Should you go into pre-term labour, particularly a very early one, the wisest thing is to get to a special unit rather than deliver in a small hospital.

Postpartum haemorrhage

At a normal delivery, a little bleeding always occurs. About a quarter of a litre is within the normal range and any healthy woman can recover this blood loss within a few days. Rarely, a bigger loss of more than half a litre of blood occurs and this could lead to serious complications unless stopped and corrected. At the time of delivery an injection is given to help the uterus contract and so stop any further blood loss. Despite this more bleeding sometimes occurs. This may be associated with retention of some membranes or a small part of the placenta. If this is so the doctor will have to remove them, usually under an anaesthetic. Were he to leave the membranes or placenta behind, the woman could bleed more heavily and thus put her life at risk. Occasionally the muscles of the uterus do not stay contracted and so the blood vessels which used to supply the placenta leak. This allows for the bleeding and needs a stronger intravenous drug treatment. Very rarely there is some damage to the neck of the womb because of the excessive stretch which occurs when the baby's head passes through; this will need repair by an obstetrician.

If the mother loses more than about one litre of blood, a blood transfusion is given. Early in the antenatal period, the blood group was checked in case of this emergency and at all properly equipped maternity units a blood bank will have stored blood of the mother's own group. Thus blood lost is replaced by that given by voluntary donors. Most women who have a postpartum haemorrhage do very well, even if they require a blood transfusion. It is difficult to predict which women will have such a bleed and so midwives give all women a uterine contracting drug at delivery. The use of this drug has reduced the incidence of postpartum haemorrhage by two-thirds and now few women die after this serious complication.

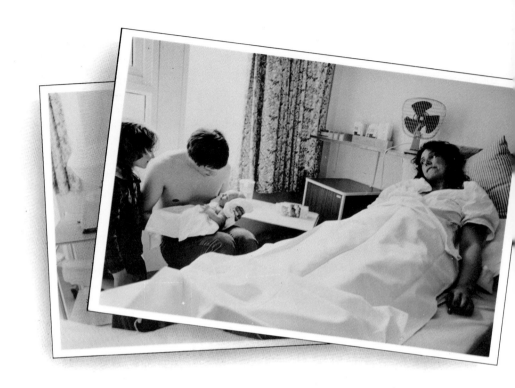

THE TIME
AFTER DELIVERY

The baby has now arrived and the high moment for which the parents have been waiting is with them. The child has been examined and pronounced normal. In the next few weeks, there is the triple task of getting the mother back to normal, learning to live with a new person in the house and dealing with the strange behaviour and feeding habits of a baby which are so different from those of an adult. Women who have had a child before at least know some of the problems that they are going to face. Those having their first baby look on the next few weeks with trepidation. Your worries may be eased if you remember that millions of the world's population have got through this phase and millions of mothers, who though anxious at first, have helped their babies grow into normal adults. You will have to observe and learn about the baby's feeding and behaviour patterns as well as watching your own body and metabolism return to their pre-pregnancy level.

CHANGES IN YOUR BODY

After the delivery is the lying-in phase. It has no precise length and does not correspond with the formal professional medical phrase, the puerperium, the time of complete recovery of the body after pregnancy—about six weeks. The lying-in phase is a much shorter time and changes with different societies at different times. Fifty years ago women lay in bed for two weeks after a normal delivery. Now they get out of bed on the same day and walk around. The lying-in period used to be considered as the time a woman stayed in hospital after delivery. This was conventionally 14 days but now most stay for about five days and some return to the care of their family doctor and community midwife in 48 hours or even on the same day as delivery. During the time after delivery, a woman's total body function and her individual organs are returning to their normal state.

The uterus

When not pregnant your uterus weighed about 60 g and was only about 8 cm long but, immediately after childbirth, it is about 30 cm long, 25 cm wide and weighs about 1 kg. Every muscle fibre is greatly elongated, being about 5 times as thick and 10 times as long. The process of returning this bulky muscular sac, which contained the baby for nine months, to the small uterus takes several weeks. Both the number and size of the muscle fibres are reduced and the blood supply is diminished. A variable amount of fibrous tissue is laid down in the walls of the uterus during this process of involution and, in consequence, the uterus will never go back quite to its pre-pregnancy state. The fibrous tissue may make its presence felt in the next pregnancy. As the uterus stretches then, so the less-elastic fibrous tissue will give a little and the woman may notice the stretch sensations of pregnancy more than she did on the first occasion.

The neck of the womb also has been changed. From the small pinpoint hole which was present before pregnancy, the cervix had to dilate up to about 10 cm diameter to allow the baby to pass. After pregnancy the neck of the womb contracts, but never achieves its pre-pregnancy state and is always a little more open. There is no harm in this for the ring of muscle lying deep beneath the mouth of the uterus is well protected in most women. The lining of the canal of the cervix may sometimes remain on the surface and lead to an area of cells known as an erosion. This is so common after a delivery that it is considered normal; most women have this area of cells for a few weeks. In the vast majority of cases, the cells retreat up the canal after a month or so and leave the surface of the cervix perfectly normal afterwards. Even those women in whom the erosion persists need not be anxious, for it is not a serious condition and does not lead to further problems of the cervix.

From the uterus comes a discharge in the days after delivery. At first, this is a vaginal loss of clots of blood and some of the thickened uterine lining which is now shed for it is no longer required. In a week or so, the colour changes from red to dark brown and then to yellow and finally to white. The losses are called the lochia and are a normal part of the process of restoration of the uterus to its pre-pregnant state. The amount and duration of lochia vary enormously in each individual. A few women have some red loss for a week after delivery, particularly if there has been a Caesarian section. This need not be a cause for concern, but you should consult your midwife if, after having faded to a yellow or white loss, the discharge again becomes bright red. Vaginal bleeding should not recur, once it has settled after childbirth, until the first proper menstrual period. Furthermore, the lochia should not be irritant or offensive; if either symptom occurs, you should contact your midwife or doctor.

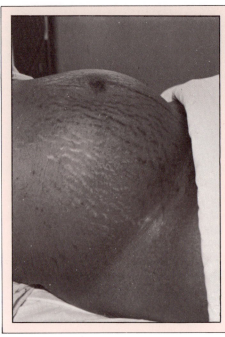

STRETCH MARKS
About one-third of pregnant women develop stretch marks. They are commonly seen in the lower stomach and less often on the thighs or breasts. They follow a sharp stretch from the underlying body and, because of a combination of a lack of elastic tissues in the skin and the hormone changes in pregnancy, the tissues just under the surface of the skin give way and a little fibrosis takes place in the gap. Unfortunately, there is little you can do to prevent them for they depend on influences you cannot control. Do not spend a lot of money on expensive creams, but massage with a simple skin cream may be of some help. When pregnancy is over, the marks often fade considerably.

The uterus before pregnancy (*right*) grows with the contained fetus to a large organ (*centre*). When delivery is over it retracts but never quite to its former size (*far right*).

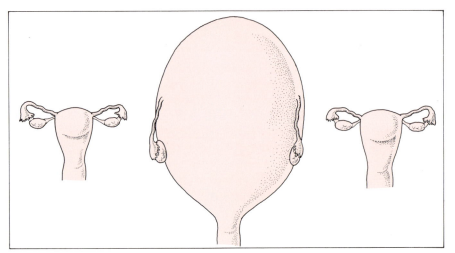

The neck of the womb (*right*) has stretched up to 10 cm to allow the baby to pass through (*centre*). After delivery, it is never quite the same: there will be a split (*far right*) rather than the original small opening.

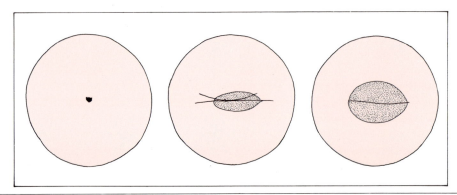

The lochia are expelled from the uterus by contractions of the uterine muscles which may be felt during the first few weeks following delivery. They can be as sharp as menstrual pains but for most women they are more of a dull ache felt in the lower stomach. Some women notice these after-pains much more when they put their baby to the breast. This is because the baby's sucking stimulates the pituitary gland to release the same hormones which are present during labour. The pains are due to the uterine contractions and usually stop a couple of weeks after delivery. Your doctor will willingly prescribe analgesics which are quite safe for you (and the baby through the breast milk) if these pains get severe.

The pelvic floor

The muscles of the vagina and supporting tissues have been stretched by childbirth. In the weeks after delivery they return to their normal state, although they will never be quite as toned up as they were before delivery. Postnatal exercises, however, can help their recovery; you should ask your midwife or physiotherapist to recommend a suitable programme of exercises.

A few women have difficulty in passing urine after childbirth. The baby's head has been stretching the pelvic tissues and may have caused some tension at the base of the bladder, leading to pain and urine retention. Occasionally a midwife may relieve this by passing a fine plastic catheter. This does not hurt but is an unusual sensation; it is well worth doing to stop the bladder stretching, a condition which could lay down problems for the future. You will pass much more urine than normal in the first few days as the body is getting rid of the extra water load collected during pregnancy. During the first 24 hours, you can pass as much as 4 or 5 litres of urine. Keep on drinking, however, to keep the flushing through effect going. After a normal delivery there is no reason why you should not go to the lavatory provided it is close by; it is much easier than balancing on hard bedpans in a curved bed in the ward.

In the first days after delivery the midwife will help you with your personal hygiene. She may suggest swabbing down the vulva and the tissues around the vagina with either a mild antiseptic solution or salt water. Many women find it comforting to use a bidet or to have a salt bath. This is an ordinary bath with about 25 cm of warm water to which you add a good fistful of kitchen (cooking) salt. This is just as beneficial as the more expensive sea salts. Sitting in a salt bath for 20 minutes twice a day will ease the ache in the perineum and help to heal a tear or episiotomy. Some women find that stitches put in for a tear or episiotomy give them pain. This should be reported to your midwife; usually it is the result of the normal healing process as the tissues knit together and will last no longer than four or five days. Very rarely problems of bruising or mild infection arise and your midwife will watch for signs of these. The stitches themselves dissolve away and mostly come out from the fifth to fifteenth day. You may find them floating in your bath as fine threads. This is quite normal for they have to be expelled. After bathing you should dry yourself gently and use sterile sanitary pads which you should change at your discretion. In the first few days after delivery the soiled pads should not be thrown away but kept for your midwife, who may wish to inspect them to check on blood loss. Discuss this point with your midwife.

The bowels

Many women have difficulty having their bowels open in the first days after delivery. No harm will result from not passing a motion for a couple of days. Probably during the day of labour not much food was taken in and so there is nothing in the pipeline to pass on. In the two or three days after this, eating is sometimes not as vigorous as normal and so again there is less material to pass on. However, after a few days you may feel uncomfortable if your bowels have not opened. Sometimes, because of the stretch of the skin of the vulva, and possibly because of the episiotomy or tear, you may worry that it may be very painful to have the bowels open. It will be more difficult if you wait for a week and then have to pass hard motions than if you manage to pass softer bulky motions in the first few days. Most doctors recommend that you take a bulky fibrous diet in the first few days to provide the bowel something to work on and to produce a soft bulky motion. Foods such as cabbage, apples or baked beans provide natural bulk. Alternatively there are proprietary fibre preparations on the market; these may be a more convenient way of building up bulk if you are not feeling very hungry. It is usually unnecessary to take

Postnatal exercises to get your body back in shape. Start the day after delivery and continue for three months. Exercises 1 and 6 strengthen the pelvic floor while the others help the abdomen.

1 Imagine that you are urinating, draw up the muscles between your legs to stop the flow. Hold for a count of four and relax.

2 With legs stretched out in front, lift your head and bend towards the right; slide your hand towards your knee. Repeat to left.

3 With knees bent, pull in your abdominal muscles; lift your head and reach with your left hand, for your right knee. Slowly lie down. Repeat to other side.

4 Raise neck and feet slightly from the floor and hold for four. Only try this if you are reasonably fit.

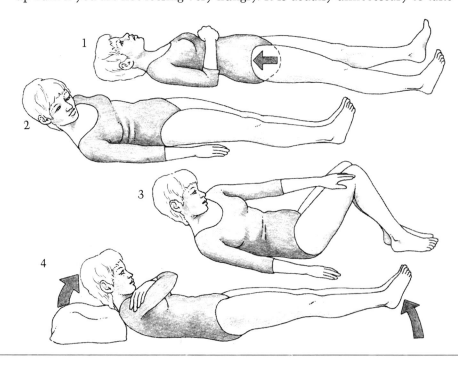

active purgatives in the time after delivery but be guided about this by your midwife. Liquid paraffin or castor oil should be avoided, although mild laxatives such as milk of magnesia or Syrup of Figs can help to establish normal bowel function in a woman who has had difficulty before, provided that there continues to be plenty of roughage in the diet.

Remember that you may also be using up extra fluids in breast feeding the baby. The bowel is the last place for the body fluids to be absorbed, and if there is extra demand on water elsewhere the motions become dehydrated and hard. This adds to the difficulty in passing them, so you should drink plenty to allow for this extra demand. Should constipation be a more difficult problem in the weeks after delivery, do not go on taking stronger purges by yourself; consult your doctor or midwife, who may be able to help you.

Emotional worries

Most women in the lying-in period have emotional disturbances. They may find themselves crying suddenly for no reason, and there may be a feeling of anticlimax after all that has happened in the months of pregnancy and the excitement of actually having the baby. Once this has taken place some of the highlights seem to be dimmed and, looking back, the delivery may not seem to be as exciting and stimulating as it was on looking forward to it. Such short attacks of mild depression, upsetting as they are, are nevertheless very common. Most women report that the excitement and happiness of looking after a new baby soon outweigh any negative feelings. Remember, too that the biochemical and hormonal changes in your body after childbirth have an effect on your thinking processes; the further away you get from childbirth the less those effects will be. Naturally, you are anxious about the new baby, as all women are; this resolves itself as you become more confident in looking after your child.

5 With knees bent, pull firmly on the abdominal muscles; lift your head, hold and relax.

6 Press the small of your back into the floor and pull on your stomach muscles as for exercise 1.

7 On your hands and knees, first arch and then hollow your back with your stomach muscles held firm.

Should these problems persist or worry you, do not hesitate to talk about them to your midwife or doctor. Your doctor is the best person to advise you which simple treatment can help postnatal blues, but the vast majority of women do not require any pharmacological assistance. Like so many things in life, time is a great healer.

The back

Among other hormonal changes in pregnancy, a great amount of progesterone is secreted into the blood. While acting specifically on the uterus, it also acts on all tissues in the body including the ligaments that support the spine. If you have a history of back trouble, there is a risk that, during pregnancy and the weeks immediately afterwards, these problems may get worse. Your increased weight and altered centre of gravity have put an extra strain on the back. Now the baby is born you can stand more upright again but, in the first days and weeks, you will spend a lot of your time looking after your new baby. This often involves leaning over him to change nappies, dress him or just to go on admiring him. Often, a mother will try to change her baby on the largest and softest surface available in the house—the double bed. This is too low and causes many women to stoop more than is good for their back. It is much wiser to look after the baby on a table or even on a shelf at chest level. Many women have a slight backache low down just above the buttocks after delivery. If this lasts more than a few days you should consult your doctor for it may be a sign of further problems in the future.

The breasts

During pregnancy, the breasts have been developing in preparation for lactation. In the last months of pregnancy, you may well have expressed clear fluid—colostrum—from the nipple. This is the preliminary to milk production. After delivery, the volume of colostrum increases for a day or two and then you will notice a tightness or distension of the breasts. From here on, proper white milk will be produced. At first there may be an over-production so that the breasts become distended and by the third or fourth day after delivery there may even be some ache or pain due to this stretch. Very soon, however, the production of milk by the breast settles to balance the removal of milk by the baby. After 7 to 10 days most women who wish to breast feed have settled into a pattern of milk production which is adequate for feeding and comfortable to make.

The breasts consist of 15 to 20 separate glandular secreting areas, all of which make milk; this is secreted along the ducts towards the nipple.

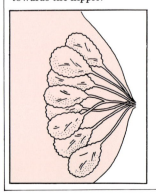

The milk is secreted in glands deep in the breast and travels up the ducts in response to the baby sucking at the nipple and the muscular action on the walls of the ducts. The hormone prolactin is produced in the mother's pituitary gland as a nervous reflex in response to the suckling and this stimulates muscular action on the wall of the ducts to produce the milk. In the first seconds of suckling the baby does not obtain much milk, but soon afterwards you notice the milk comes at a rush.

During the time that you are learning to feed your baby and your baby is learning to feed from you, the midwife is a crucial friend. She has seen breast feeding before with all its variations. No two women are the same and she can be a valuable aide to guide you in this normal aspect of life. It is sometimes very aggravating at first if the baby does not fix on or if you do not seem to make enough milk, but, with patience, most women can feed their babies for

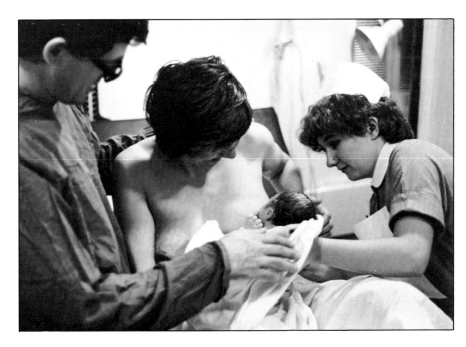

Soon after delivery, the baby may wish to try a feed. There is no milk at this stage, but it is immensely satisfying to both mother and child.

as long as they want to. Remember, it is a new method of feeding for the baby and he too needs to learn. In the UK about 70 per cent of women now breast feed their children while the rest use bottle formulae. See pages 159 to 164 for further information on infant feeding.

ROLE OF THE FATHER

The time immediately after childbirth is a critical one in family life. You are over the high of pregnancy and childbirth and now you have the tiring job of looking after the newborn baby. Your partner should try to take time off work so that he can contribute more to the family at this stage; this will help to bond him to you and to his new baby, as well as offering you some relief from domestic chores. You will want all the help you can get at this time so that you can do what, for the moment, you are best at—looking after the newborn baby. You will also want a lot of care and affection for emotions swing widely during this time of potential stress.

If the baby is not being breast fed, then the father can very quickly learn to bottle feed the child just as well as the mother. He can help prepare feeds and take turns with the actual feeding. He may wake and share the night work, for there is nothing more frustrating for a woman than sitting up at three o'clock in the morning soothing and feeding a crying infant with a husband snoring alongside. If you are breast feeding, then your partner may like to sit with you and provide companionship.

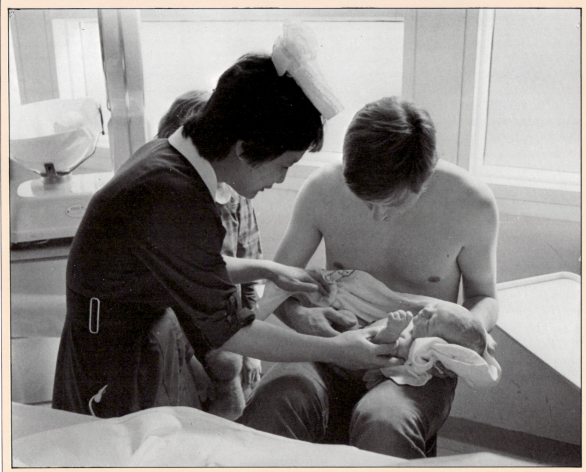

When a baby is born he belongs to the whole family. The mother may have done the work, but the father and other children will want to get to know the new baby very soon.

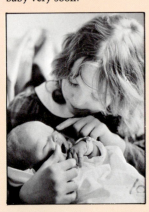

INVOLVING THE REST OF THE FAMILY

Increasingly in the last weeks of pregnancy, during labour and in the first days after delivery, your mind will have been concentrated on the new baby. Other children in the family may have noticed this. You and your partner must overcompensate and ensure that the children do not feel left out for they do not always understand the excitement to you of the new family member. Try to prepare your children for the new baby right from the beginning of your pregnancy even before the swelling in your stomach is obvious. Children are very observant and will notice that you are getting fatter. Let the children come to the antenatal clinic with you and give them every opportunity to examine your growing bump. If they are old enough, let them listen to the baby and feel the movements inside. They will be intrigued.

Very soon after delivery, introduce the newborn baby to the other children in the family. Let them handle him and, provided they are in good health, let them hold him with reasonable safety measures. Involve the other children as much as possible in looking after the baby so they do not feel left out. Try to spend time during the day specifically with the other children and away from the baby to show that you care for them.

PROFESSIONAL HELP

After childbirth, particularly if it is your first baby, professional help is there for you to use when you need it. In the hospital there are qualified midwives on duty 24 hours a day. It is remarkable how problems which would not trouble you by daylight may loom menacingly at two o'clock in the morning, and a friendly talk with a midwife may reassure you about many otherwise minor points. The medical staff in the hospital will make regular rounds and see you at their visits to the ward, usually at least once a day. Should you have a problem, do not hesitate to call the midwife; if necessary, she will contact the doctor, who will come according to the degree of urgency.

In the first 24 hours, your baby will have been examined by one of the obstetricians or by a pediatrician. This is the first formal examination of the child's life. In the labour ward, the obstetrician or midwife would have checked the baby briefly for external signs of problems and to ensure that breathing is well established. Most of the problems are excluded by such a brief examination but the more formal physical examination goes further than this. First of all the doctor looks at the attitude in which the child is lying, that he is relaxed with the limbs gently flexed on to the body. The baby's colour is examined to see that there is good oxygenation and no anaemia or jaundice. Starting at the head, the pediatrician will check the skull to see that

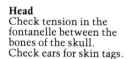
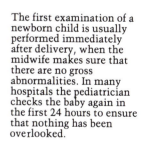

Head
Check tension in the fontanelle between the bones of the skull. Check ears for skin tags.

Face
Check eyes for degree of slant. Check upper lip for notching. Check hard palate for any deficiency.

Chest
Check heart for gross abnormal murmurs. Check lungs for adequate air entry on each side.

Stomach
Check umbilicus for number of blood vessels — there should be two arteries and one vein. Check hernial sites in groins for any protrusion.

Genitals
Female — inspect but do not part. Male — check scrotal sac for one testicle descended into each side. Check penis for orifice on tip.

The first examination of a newborn child is usually performed immediately after delivery, when the midwife makes sure that there are no gross abnormalities. In many hospitals the pediatrician checks the baby again in the first 24 hours to ensure that nothing has been overlooked.

Hands
Check fingers for extra digits. Check palms for creases.

Back
Check for any deficiency in the bony spine. Check for hair patches in the lower back.

Hips
Check hips for normal articulation in their sockets.

Knees
Check articulation of joints with no overextension.

Ankles
Check flexibility of the joints and exclude club feet. Check number of toes.

the bones and the lines at which they join are normal; the ears are inspected to see that there are no extra skin tags. The face is examined for any cleft in the palate and the eyes (externally) to ensure that the lid system is normal. There is no point in flashing bright lights into the baby's eyes at this stage. The sucking reflex of the mouth is checked also by slipping a little finger in between the gums. The chest is examined with a stethoscope to listen to the heart sounds. These are faster than an adult's and usually two distinct sounds can be heard at each beat. The doctor will also want to listen for any murmurs that might indicate a problem heart; these are rare. The bases of the lungs will also be checked to make sure that the air entry into these organs is good.

Examination of the stomach follows; the umbilical cord remnant will be checked to see that it is dry and not in any way infected. The groins are inspected for hernias which, although rare, do happen at this stage of life. The bottom is usually checked but by this time most babies will have passed early stools, so it will be obvious that there is no obstruction. Further, the midwife will have slipped a thermometer into the bottom to check the baby's temperature soon after delivery. This is another test to make sure there is no obstruction. The external genital organs are examined. In a girl, the pediatrician will merely check the lips of the vagina and look at the clitoris. The lips of the vagina are not spread apart, nor is there any internal examination. In a boy, it is essential to check that there is one testicle in each side of the scrotum even if it may be a little high up in the sac. The penis will be examined to make sure that the orifice for passing water is towards the tip, for the direction of the stream depends upon this later in life.

BIRTH REGISTRATION

It is the legal requirements for all babies' births to be notified to a registrar of births and deaths within six weeks of the event (in Scotland three weeks). In some hospitals registrars visit on regular days during the week, so you can do this registration while you are in the lying-in phase. However, with economies in the social services these visits have been cut in many areas and you may have to go to the registrar's office. The hospital can tell you the nearest one to your home. Usually one of the parents registers the birth, although it could be done in exceptional cases by the person who delivered the child or the person in charge of the obstetric unit (in Scotland a relative of either parent can perform this task). The details a registrar requires are the date and place of birth, the sex of the child and each parent's name and place of birth. They will also ask about the father's occupation. If the couple is not married then the occupation of the child's father is only asked for with the assent of both parties. The last item may seem a strange detail to include, but those involved in planning such things as schooling and employment needs use birth data to identify different socio-economic groups in the population. The first name of the child is not required at this stage so do not worry if you have not yet agreed a name.

You will receive free from the registrar a short birth certificate which has the basic information about your child—name, sex, date and place of birth. Later on, when the birth has been coded on central computers of the Office of Population and Census Surveys you can apply for a full certificate for a small fee.

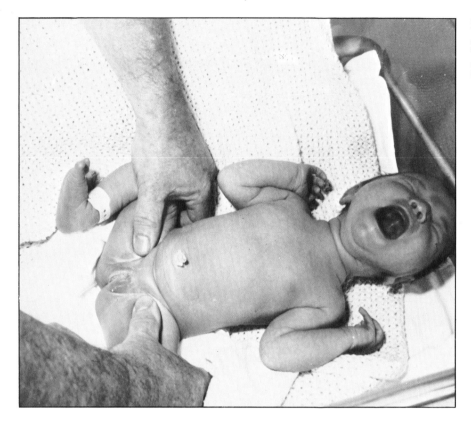

One of the problems the baby may have is dislocation of the hips. This can be checked quite simply by the test shown here.

The limbs will be examined, the arms and hands inspected to make sure there are no extra digits and that the fingers are normally formed. The hips are checked to make sure there is no looseness of hip joint and no dislocation. The knees and feet are checked to ensure that the ankle joints are not turned in or out and finally the toes are inspected.

After this examination, which takes about five minutes, the pediatrician will be able to assure you that you have a normal child. Certainly there could be one or two abnormalities that are deep inside the baby showing no signs; they cannot be detected for weeks, months or years and are only known about and can only be treated in adult life. These are very rare and should not be considered now.

Members of the team

While in the delivery room and the ward, you will meet an array of doctors, midwives and other professionals. The obstetricians are obviously the doctors making decisions about the pregnancy. They work with anaesthetists who provide the epidurals and, if necessary, general anaesthesia. An essential member of the team that looks after you both is the pediatrician. If it is thought early on that there might be a problem with your baby you may have met this doctor already. He will willingly discuss with you the implications of any conditions diagnosed after birth. Increasingly inside the hospital, the pediatrician is becoming involved with antenatal care and is commonly the person in the labour ward if difficulties with the baby occur or are even suspected. Any large maternity unit will have a pediatrician on duty in the

Grades of midwife can often be distinguished by their uniform. Dark blue is worn by a sister and light blue by trained staff midwives — the colour of the belt indicates seniority. The white uniform is worn by a nursery nurse whose primary duties are to look after the babies and help the mothers in their bathing and feeding.

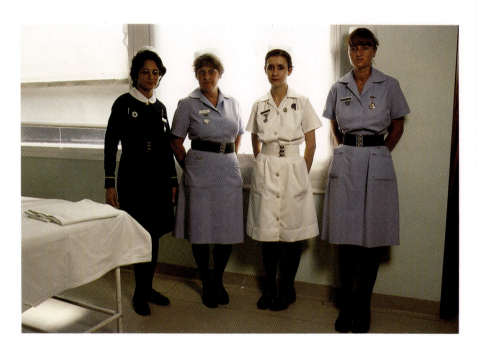

hospital all the time for potential problems. After delivery, the pediatrician usually performs examinations on the normal child and advises the mother about any problems that arise. The pediatrician will be the professional specialist who will care for the medical needs of your child for the next 15 years. It is essential that the pediatrician is involved early in the child's life so that he can get to know the child and carry on through. In British medical practice, much of the pediatric work outside the hospital is performed by the GP who is usually skilled in the care of children. When he is in difficulty he may refer the child to a specialist pediatrician at the hospital.

The midwives and nurses in the hospital wear uniforms which differ in style from one unit to another but all commonly indicate in some way the seniority of that staff member. Other professionals may well be involved in the mother's care. The medical social worker may have seen the woman during pregnancy to help with social problems that she or her family have. If these continue afterwards she will, of course, continue her care throughout the puerperium and she usually works both inside the hospital and in the community. The physiotherapist may have met the mother at antenatal classes and will probably see her in the lying-in ward after delivery where she helps with the physical restoration of the body.

When you leave hospital and go home, you will be visited by midwives from the community service. These may be the same women as the hospital team, taking their turn on the rota. If you have been delivered by a GP and community midwife then of course that team will look after you in the home. The midwife visits every day for the first 10 days after delivery to help with problems and check mother and baby's health. If required, she will continue visiting for 28 days after childbirth. The health visitor will start her visits to the home before the midwife has finished her responsibility so that there is continuous care. If, as is the case in some districts, the health visitor is associated with both the GP antenatal clinic and the hospital clinic, you are likely to know her already. The health visitor will then be the link between the mother and the GP in the early days of the child's life and she will help to see that all goes smoothly.

WHAT TO EAT

Immediately after delivery it is unlikely you will be thinking much about food. You may well be thirsty and traditionally, in Britain, cups of tea for mother and father are one of the first requisites after delivery. Do not forget that the baby also may be thirsty so, if you are going to breast feed, the first minutes after delivery is a great time to start the child getting used to the habit.

In the days that follow delivery, you will probably want to drink a lot and this is quite normal. The amount you eat is likely to be very variable. Some women do not feel like eating immediately after childbirth but they should ensure that enough bulk gets into the body to allow the bowels to work normally. When the restorative changes that we have already described are taking place in the body, it is wise to follow a well-planned diet to help lay down new tissues. If breast feeding, you will require even more nutrition and extra fluid to make up for what is lost in the milk. While appetites vary, the principles of a balanced diet which were followed in pregnancy should be continued into the time after delivery. In hospital, the diets may be a little bleak as NHS hospitals have a very limited sum of money to spend on diet and it is difficult to housekeep attractively on such minute finances. You may wish to have extras brought in by your partner; cheeses, fresh fruit and yogurts all help. You may well be loaded with chocolates and sweets by well-meaning friends. Share those with the other people in the ward for they are not so useful as the body-building foods.

If you are breast feeding you must remember that when the habit is fully established you can be providing more than a litre of milk a day to the infant. This represents about 700 calories, so to continue to breast feed successfully you need the extra food and fluid in amounts equal to an increase of about a

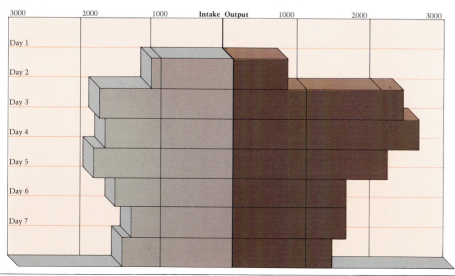

In the days immediately after delivery, the kidneys excrete more water than is taken in. During pregnancy excess fluid will have built up in the blood and must now be shed.

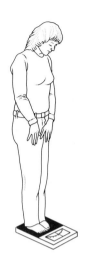

After the baby is born, it is hard to lose weight, but check your weight once a week to make sure that you are not gaining.

quarter in most women's normal food intake and fluid requirements. This need can probably be met by drinking about half a litre of cow's milk a day and slightly increasing the amount of protein (body-building foods) you eat. If you dislike milk there is no necessity for you to take your extra protein in this way, it is simply quite convenient for those who do. The details of the constituents of human breast milk have been well worked out by your body. They are not specifically related to what you eat or do not eat, except in cases of extreme starvation. However, certain foods do go across in breast milk and may affect the child; in particular curries and rhubarb are known to cause problems. Watch carefully for any particular food to which your baby reacts and avoid it. Generally speaking, with ordinary intake, most foods have no effect on the baby.

Continue the good diet habits you started in pregnancy. Eat plenty of protein and do not eat excess carbohydrate. The time of looking after a child is one when you cannot concentrate much on yourself or your figure; if you overeat carbohydrates at this stage, weight can go on which is difficult to remove later. It is almost impossible to diet during this phase of life but at least you need not increase excessively. Stand on the scales once a week, to ensure that you are not putting on too much weight. Do not weigh daily for this does not give you a good general picture, you are merely seeing the trees and not the wood.

RESTARTING WORK

Childbirth is a time of acutely hard physical work. Pregnancy is a time of chronic physical work. You need, therefore, a period to recover from both of these, however fit and well you are. It is sensible not to return to ordinary work immediately after delivery. The exact time for this will vary enormously from one woman to another. Obviously, work involving less manual effort could be started before heavy activity. If you have a job which requires concentrated thought, remember that after childbirth your capacity to concentrate is temporarily diminished by the hormone changes in your body, and you may not produce your best work at this time. Fatigue due to night feeding adds to this, so do not plan to go back to work too soon even if you feel quite strong enough to do so.

Most women find that by about six weeks after delivery they are ready for moderate activity but this is not an absolute figure and varies greatly. It is impossible to lay down rules; social security benefits start for most women at 28 weeks and continue until 7 weeks after delivery and it is probably best to take advantage of this. However, you should be guided by your own feelings. If you wish to start some activity, try it; if it does not hurt you or tire you, then by all means continue. However, if either of these symptoms occurs you are not yet ready for starting that particular work.

PROBLEMS THAT MAY ARISE

Most women have a normal time after delivery enjoying looking after their baby. However, in a few cases problems can arise. We have already considered some of these but a few are potentially more serious unless professional aid is obtained quickly.

Infection

The uterus is particularly susceptible to infection after delivery, for there is a large raw area where the placenta was attached. Infection may show itself by pain and an offensive discharge from the vagina accompanied by a raised temperature. Treatment, if properly given, resolves the problem quickly and so you should report any symptoms to your midwife.

Urinary tract infections usually show up as pain on passing water and again a raised temperature. Let your doctors know; they can check and give you treatment quickly.

It is rare to get a breast infection these days but, if you do, it will be a sore area localized to one quadrant of the breast. It may throb, and prompt treatment is required. Mild breast infections need not stop you breast feeding from the other breast, but the milk from the affected breast should not be used for it may contain bacteria. It can be hand expressed and discarded.

Thrombosis

After pregnancy the blood is in a state which makes it more likely to clot in the veins. This is made worse by any sluggishness of circulation and for this reason women are encouraged to leave their bed and exercise their legs early after delivery. A clot in the leg usually shows as an acutely painful area in the calf, below and behind the knee. Report this to your midwife immediately; prompt treatment can prevent more serious complications arising.

Bleeding

Most women have lochia (see pages 141 to 143) which pale in colour as the days go by. If, however, bright red bleeding from the vagina should return, report this for it may need prompt attention.

THE POSTNATAL VISIT

About six weeks after delivery, it is wise to have a check up. By this time most of the organs will have reached their resting state and you should be well established into feeding your baby by whatever method you choose. If you have delivered at hospital, you may return to the postnatal clinic there or you might visit your own doctor. If your GP delivered you, he will certainly do the postnatal examination.

When you are seen at the postnatal visit, the professionals will check your health. You will be weighed and your blood pressure will be checked again now. If you are breast feeding, your breasts will be checked and you can discuss your feeding. An examination of the stomach reveals how the tone of the muscles is going . An internal examination will reveal if the uterus has gone back to its normal size and the neck of the womb is well healed. Often a cervical smear is taken at this time in order to ensure that the neck of the womb has no disease. This is a part of your general health check and prevention of illness; it is wise to have such a smear done every few years.

An important part of the postnatal visit is discussion of contraception. If you have not done so already, you should take the opportunity of considering this with your advisers. Contraception is free in this country and you should consider the methods described in Chapter 9 to find one that suits you.

The puerperium is a busy time. The baby is getting used to the parents and the parents to the baby. The new member of the family demands a lot of time and physical effort but, although tiring, this is very rewarding. The simple measures outlined in this section may help you enjoy this time better.

A small speculum can be inserted into the vagina so that the neck of the womb can be seen. A wooden spatula then allows a cervical smear to be taken.

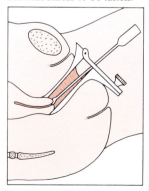

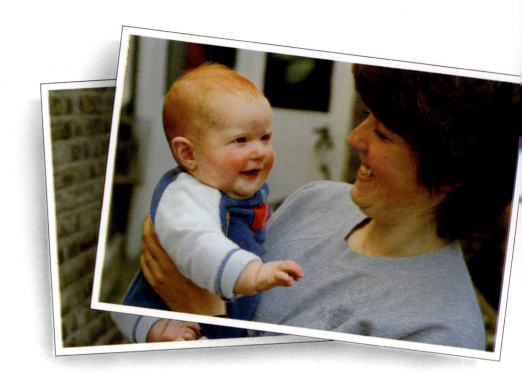

THE NEWBORN CHILD

The hard work of labour is over, the midwife has tidied things up and you have now taken over the baby to whom you have looked forward for many months. You and your partner have now got the child who is going to occupy your thoughts and physical efforts for the next few years. He or she (and with no chauvinism, but for the sake of editorial ease we will refer to the newborn baby as he, as elsewhere in the book) has developed in the uterus to a certain stage of growth but he is still immature.

NEWBORN ACTIVITY

Babies differ in their ability to cope with the external world according to the stage of pregnancy at which they are delivered. A baby born at full term (40 weeks gestation from the first day of the last normal menstrual period) is capable of sustaining respiration, once started, of maintaining circulation of blood around the body and of coping with a compatible temperature environment. He could not support himself if sat up but he can move his limbs very actively. If you put your index finger across his palm he will grasp it tightly, a reflex surviving from our primate ancestors whose newborn infants needed it to hang on to their mothers or to the branches of trees in which they lived.

He can usually smell and he is particularly fast at learning the smell of his own mother's breast milk which he can distinguish from that of another woman by about a week after delivery. Vision is not well focused at first, but this ability follows in a few weeks. Immediately after birth, his eyes will follow moving objects and he seems to prefer some patterns rather than others; for example he will prefer looking at the shape of a face rather than a blank pattern. If you get him to look at you and then put out your tongue, he will probably copy this and he will show signs of listening when talked to. He cannot move his head very well but can move his eyes. If you hold your baby just above a firm surface he will make distinct walking steps in sequence. The earlier that a baby is born before full term the less well developed he is, so the more he will depend upon your support and upon professional outside help. Life depends upon the ability of the central nervous system (the brain and spinal cord) to keep the blood pressure steady in the body and to balance heat production against heat loss, so stabilizing the internal temperature. The heart must go on beating and respiration must continue its rhythm of breathing in and out. The earlier a child is born into the world the less developed is the central nervous system and so the more these various functions may need assistance. In the last weeks of life in the uterus, fat is laid down including the layers under the skin. It is this that gives the newborn child his round, chubby look. Should he be born before this padding-up process can occur, he will look very scrawny and the mother may consider him to be malnourished, but weight-gain can be very rapid. In the first days after birth you will be enthralled with what your baby can do.

Sleeping

It is said in many of the-books-that-advise-mothers that babies sleep for most of the time. This unhelpful advice then worries those mothers whose babies have not read these books, for some babies sleep a lot less than others. Provided the baby is contented, this does not matter and the newborn child may lie with eyes open, gently making sucking motions with his lips. If you have a baby who sleeps a lot except when being fed, this is very convenient, for it allows you to press on with other activities in between feeds. Other babies, however, have a series of short sleeps and wake up in between. Do not automatically assume that the baby is hungry in these intervals, it may be just that his brain is working and he wakes up after a short sleep. Some babies drift off to sleep, others go suddenly. Some wake up with a jerk, others just open their eyes and seem to go from the sleeping to the waking state with no transitional phase. The child who is hungry will soon make his presence known. The child who is not hungry, but awake, will just lie there contentedly with his mind in neutral.

Crying

A baby's cry can be a sign of great consolation to the mother and father immediately after he is born. It shows he has taken enough air into the lungs and is now expelling it through the vocal cords and so is an independent air-breathing human being. From then on, crying can assume an enormous problem in the minds of some parents; they associate crying with more adult reactions and think the baby must be unhappy or in pain. To the child, crying is merely a form of breathing out, and his only means of communication.

Babies do have temperamental differences and some are more irritable than others. The personality of a newborn baby often reflects the behaviour

The baby can see a lot. If you make faces at him, he will copy them.

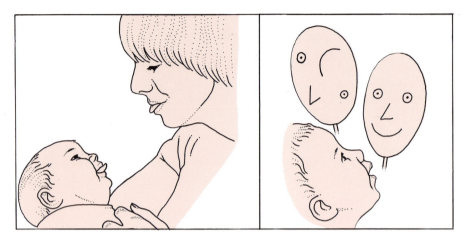

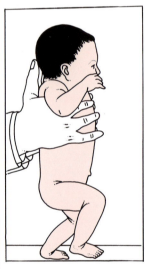

If you support your baby over a firm surface, he will make walking movements within a few days of birth.

pattern of the child later in life. You will need to observe your own baby's patterns of sleeping and crying, for each individual has a different reaction to the new environment. Remember the enormous differences between life inside the uterus and the existence outside. The former is a relatively quiet, warm, dark life with no effort needed to breathe or take in food, both of which were supplied automatically by the placenta. After birth, the baby must very quickly get used to a bright, noisy and cool world where breathing must be established in a few minutes and feeding in a few days. No wonder he is perplexed and sometimes uncertain.

Some of the more obvious causes of excessive crying in a baby can be watched for and remedied. For instance, in warm weather the baby may be sweating a little and may cry because he is thirsty. If you offer some water from a bottle between feeds he will soon gulp this down. This will often stop the baby crying. Similarly, some babies cry at first when they pass urine. This is a sudden cry which usually lasts a few moments only.

More repetitive is the cry of colic as the child's large bowel works on simple motions or gas passing through the loops of bowel. With recurrent bouts of crying, the child pulls up his legs and tenses himself; often the episode is relieved by a very audible sound of wind passing. The simpler forms of colic are best treated by picking the child up and carrying him over your shoulder or rocking him. Parents may find that it helps to put the child in the pram and wheel him around so that the movements soothe; sometimes a long drive in the back seat of a car does the trick. Check that the feeding does not contain any colic-making substances such as curry; make sure that the baby is not taking too much air at the same time as milk. Many of the commercial gripe mixtures bought in the chemist's shop help different babies and it is worth trying them. Should colic still continue consult your doctor or midwife.

Newborn children can cry from loneliness or from tiredness if they have missed a sleep. Hunger crying usually follows a gap since the last meal but do not believe the books-that-advise-mothers that this only happens every four hours. It can happen two hourly or even more frequently and you may need to offer him the breast or a bottle more often than four hourly. Do not become a slave to his demands in this, but see if you can space the feeds out a

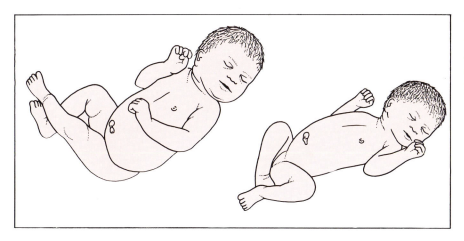

A baby born preterm is scrawny (*right*) compared with the one who comes out at the right time (*left*). Fat layers are laid down in the last weeks of pregnancy and these are missing from the preterm baby.

little in order to allow you some time to do other things between feeding. At first your child may need as many as 12 or as few as 6 feeds a day and you must find the right pattern. Over the weeks, you can gradually alter this to lengthen the interval between feeds.

Crying may indicate some illness. The baby may be feverish, there may be some vomiting or diarrhoea, or there may be more severe pain in the stomach indicated by a drawing up of the legs. If this continues for longer than a normal short attack of colic, and if it does not stop even when the baby is picked up and comforted, you should consult your doctor, midwife or health visitor.

Feeding the baby

Newborn mammals are fed on milk. Natural evolution has made sure that the best milk to feed mammal babies with is that of their own species, and so breast feeding your baby is almost certainly the best way to feed him. Until this century artificial milks were not available. If a woman was unable to feed her own child, she employed another woman, who was still making milk, to feed her baby, and records exist of wet nurses, as they were called, taking on as many as six infants and going on lactating for several years. If a wet nurse could not be found, the child commonly died. Artificial milk feeding came in this century; the preparations are mostly made from dried cow's milk powder to which are added various supplements to make up for the lack of iron and vitamins. These are added to water to make a mixture which approximates to breast milk. However, it often does not make up the balanced nourishment which breast milk provides. Nor can it provide the better protection that maternal antibodies give the newborn baby in the first weeks of life. These antibodies can prevent intestinal and respiratory infection and possibly protect also against some of the allergic problems like eczema and asthma. Undoubtedly the constituents of human breast milk are best suited to absorption from the human baby's intestine. Artificially made milk must be made to the correct concentration directed on the package. If not, the baby might receive too much of certain minerals, particularly sodium and phosphate, and these can cause harm. It is much easier to overfeed a baby with artificial milk and make him too heavy.

One of the problems of breast feeding is that only one person can feed and you may not be available if you are at work or if the milk production is reduced when you are ill. Most women actually enjoy breast feeding, and yet many say that bottle feeding can be just as enjoyable for the child is held equally close for both methods. At least with bottle feeding your partner can give you a hand and so relieve you of some of your tasks — at the same time he will experience for himself some of the pleasure of feeding the baby.

Some women are afraid that breast feeding alters the shape of the breasts making them larger or a little heavier. This is not so. The changes that occur in the breasts are due to pregnancy itself and not to anything that happens afterwards. The breasts of a woman who has breast fed are no different from those who have bottle fed.

Breast feeding

The baby can start breast feeding soon after he is delivered; many have their first feed before leaving the labour ward. The milk produced at this time is thin and called colostrum. It has protein and carbohydrate in it but little fat and so does not look as opaque and white as ordinary milk; it is, however, highly concentrated and very good for the baby, and is quite enough for him without any extra feeding.

After about three days the more conventionally expected milk comes in, often rather speedily and in excess. This causes filling of the breasts and distension can be painful. The baby will relieve most of this but some women require a little help to get rid of the surplus. Eventually, milk-making settles down to an even balance; the baby removes the amount he needs with the breasts making only that amount each day. Suckling the baby at the breast is the best method of ensuring regular production.

It is important that you and your baby are in the right position when you breast feed. You should be sitting well supported in a firm upright chair with a good back so that you can take the baby in one arm, supporting his head with the elbow. Ensure that when the baby goes to the breast he can breathe through his nose. He will usually take the nipple right into his mouth and his gums will actually engage on the dark areas of the skin around the nipple. In this way he will massage the milk out of the nipple rather than suck it; if you allow him to suck too hard the nipple may become sore. While the first few feeds may be frustrating to both you and the baby, eventually he will get the message and will start strong regular sucking.

In the first week of life the baby will lose some weight due to a loss of water from his body. This is quite normal and does not indicate that he is not getting enough milk. By the end of the first week, feeding should be matching demand with supply. In these early days, the breast can leak a little milk between the feeds. This can be a nuisance and nursing pads must be worn inside the nursing bra to prevent it staining the clothing. Change the pads frequently, for wet pads irritate the skin of the nipples.

Most women who breast feed let the baby feed when he wants to. This demand feeding can be very frequent at first but usually settles down to every three or four hours. At night most babies still demand a feed every three or four hours and this can be a very tiring business. With breast feeding there is only one person to do it but your partner could be helpful by getting up and making a cup of tea and talking to you while the breast feeding is going on. It is

Milk is made in glands deep inside the breasts. When the baby starts to suck on the nipple this stimulates the mother to release the hormone prolactin. This acts on the muscles of the walls of the ducts and milk is gently propelled towards the nipple.

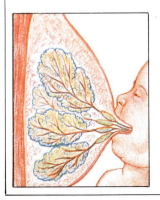

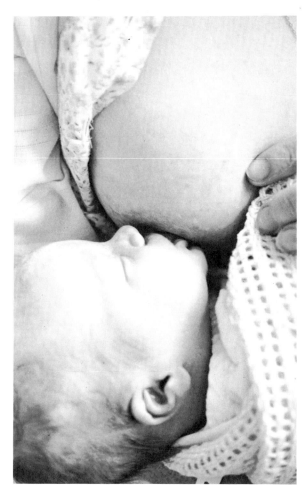

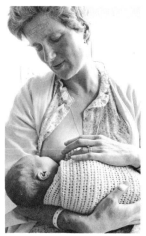

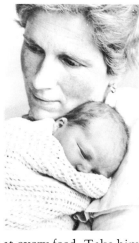

The pleasure a woman gets from breast feeding her baby is obvious. These pictures show that the baby's satisfaction is considerable too.

probably wise to let the baby feed from each breast at every feed. Take him from the first breast while he is still actively sucking and start on the second, where he will finish off the feed. It is probably sensible (if you can remember) to start feeding on alternate breasts each time. Do not become enslaved to these suggestions; follow then when you remember but much more importantly *relax*. Relaxation is the real key to successful breast feeding.

If you have twins it is quite possible to breast feed. Milk is made in ample amounts but it will take much more time to manage the trick of feeding both babies simultaneously. It will help if you can find someone who has had experience to show you how. The NCT or Twins Association may be able to put you in touch with someone who can help. It is difficult if one of the babies needs attention in the middle of the feeding period because then the other will have to be put down, but more often, breast feeding twins can be made to work.

There are few medical reasons why a woman should not breast feed. Certain drugs may go through the breast milk and affect the child. If a woman is on such long-term treatment she may be asked to discontinue. Some women who have chronic debilitating diseases may not be able to continue but women with diabetes can breast feed quite happily.

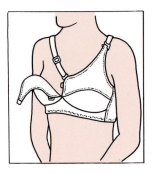
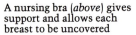
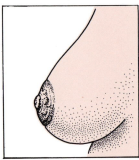
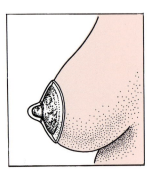

A nursing bra (*above*) gives support and allows each breast to be uncovered

separately. A flattened or inverted nipple (*above*) can make feeding difficult. You

can use a plastic shield during feeding if the nipple remains flat (above).

Occasionally an infection of the breast occurs; in such cases it would be wise to stop feeding from the infected breast because of bacteria in the milk which could affect the baby. This breast may be hand expressed to remove any excess milk and the baby fed from the other side until the infection is cured, when full feeding can recommence.

Bottle feeding

About one third of the women in this country bottle feed their infants. The bottle, made of plastic or glass, has a cap with a rubber teat on top through which the child sucks milk. He should be held in the same way as for breast feeding; he must be comfortable and his mouth should be held higher than the stomach.

The milk should be prepared precisely according to the instructions given on the packet or tin. It is not a good idea to give a little more of the powder in order to give more nutrients to the child. Boiled water which has been allowed to cool is the best solvent and the eventual mix should be just warm when given to the child. There is no merit in giving hot milk to a baby and the temperature should be checked on your wrist before the child takes it. The milk is at the right temperature when it feels neither hot nor cold when squirted on to the inside of your wrist. This means that it is at blood heat. Do ensure that the equipment is clean and not a source of bacterial infection. Bottles and teats must be washed carefully, and stored in a mild antiseptic solution such as Milton.

DEMAND FEEDING

Feeding the baby soon falls into a pattern. Some try to organize it by the clock, feeding the child every so many hours; others use demand feeding, providing feed when the baby demands it (and such demands can be very vocative). The former may be convenient for the mother but is over-regimentation. The latter is more pleasant but time-consuming; whichever you start with, you will end up doing the same thing, feeding your child every two-and-a-half to four hours.

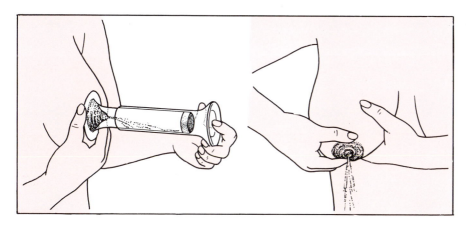

Milk may be expressed by means of a breast pump (*far left*) or by massaging the breast by hand (*left*). Massage takes more practice, however, than using a pump.

The best way of starting bottle feeding is to get the child interested. Gently stroke his cheek and, as he turns his head and purses his lips, place the moistened teat against them; he will take the teat deep into his mouth and feed. Babies have different patterns of feeding. Some will take the whole feed in one go, others pause and leave some of the bottle behind. This is all part of normal human variation, although small babies may well take much more than very large ones. The amount offered at each feed should be based upon the volume that most children will want; this is usually 85 ml for each half kilogram of their weight every 24 hours. Thus it can be divided into the number of feeds a day the child is going to have. Hence a 3 kg baby requires about 6 x 85 or 510 ml in 24 hours. If he is offered every six hours, mix 85ml at each feed. Very small children require more frequent feeds than larger ones.

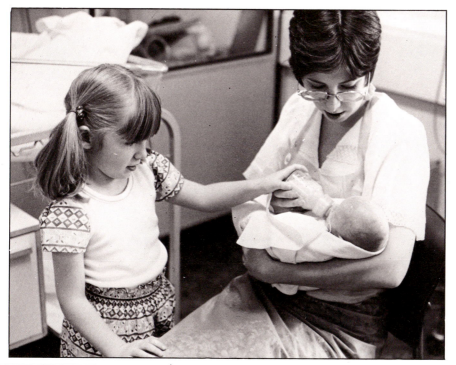

Bottle feeding (*left*) can be emotionally satisfying too. One great advantage is that other members of the family can join in and lend a hand.

It is important that the equipment used for bottle feeding is kept scrupulously clean and sterile. Any small amount of milk left behind can act as a focus of bacteriological infection and can lead to gastro-intestinal illness in the child.

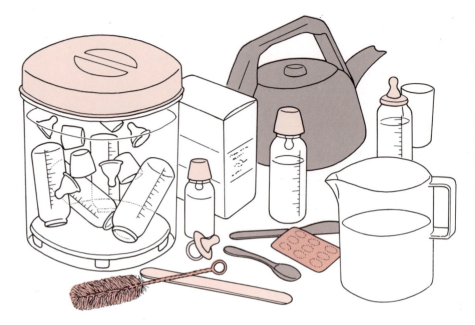

The best guide to whether the child is getting enough is that the child is both happy and contented and that there is steady weight gain. Of these guidelines, the baby's behaviour rather than his weight gain is the better measure.

A baby takes in air which he swallows during feeding and this happens more from the bottle than the breast. A bubble gathers in the stomach and can be uncomfortable. The baby should therefore be sat up over your shoulder and his back massaged with a mixture of rubbing and mild thumping movements in order to help him break wind. He will be much more comfortable after that. Some babies need this after every feed and a few need it in the middle of a feed.

Problems that may arise

Most babies lead a contented life, not worrying the parents unduly. However, some symptoms may arise and, whatever they may be, they are always a worry, particularly if it is your first baby. One major concern many parents have is when to call in a doctor, midwife or health visitor. If you are worried about a child no professional ever minds being contacted. The major symptoms are that:

he is not fully conscious
he has had a fever fit
he becomes pale or is blue around the lips and face
he has difficulty in breathing or appears to be wheezing
a sudden rash appears

All of these should alert you to get medical help immediately. The other symptoms that we will discuss are usually of a milder nature and can be coped with by less urgent consultations.

Vomiting

Many babies bring up a little milk at the end of a feed while they are being winded. This is normal; others have frequent small vomits during the day — a sign often that winding has not been complete. Providing he is contented and gaining weight this is not serious. Should the child have a large vomit, losing most of the feed, particularly if this comes back with some force, then the doctor should be consulted in case this is a sign of infection or obstruction.

Many children get a mild pain as their bowel contracts upon the food going through it. When living in the uterus, there was nothing passing down the bowel and so no work was required. Within a few days of birth it has to learn how to propel the solids on and many babies reflect this new use of the bowel by waves of colic, particularly in the early evening and in the middle of the night. They cry, hold their breath, go red in the face, curl their legs up on to their stomach and go rigid. Providing this lasts only some seconds it is a sign that the bowel is learning to deal with the contained solid. Many of the proprietary gripe mixtures are of help. Since each one contains a different calminative it is probably sensible to try more than one before giving them up. If colic persists, you should consult your doctor who may prescribe something stronger to help the muscles of the intestine to relax.

Colic

Most babies gain weight but the range is very variable. If there is persistent lack of weight gain so that the infant's weight is dropping well below the normal range for his age, you should consult the doctor or health visitor. This, however, does not apply in the first week of life when a slight weight loss is normal.

Poor weight gain

The most common reason for constipation in babies is lack of fluid. This leads to the stools becoming dry and hard, and difficult to pass. However, do not consider that a baby has to empty his bowels every day. Remember that milk does not contain very many solid constituents and much of that taken in is absorbed into the body, so there is little left to pass on. This applies particularly to breast milk. If you are concerned, extra water may be given to the baby particularly in warm weather.

Constipation

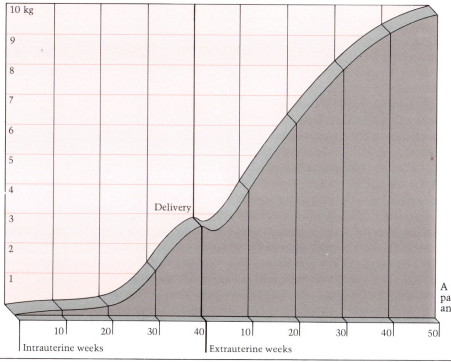

A typical weight-gain pattern for a child before and after delivery.

Diarrhoea	Loose watery motions on the nappy may mean that the child has an infection and one should watch carefully for other signs, such as fever, sweating or flushing. Sometimes, however, a simpler solution is obvious. The mother may be taking a cascara type laxative which goes through the breast milk to the baby. In rarer cases, there may be variations of absorption of sugar by the child in the gut and so the motions are very loose.
Fever fits	Very rarely a newborn child gets a high temperature due to infecton and has a seizure. The baby goes into a fugue, becomes stiff and then starts to twitch his limbs. This lasts for a few seconds and, following recovery, he drifts off to sleep. Such seizures are unusual in newborn babies but, when they occur, they are nearly always due to a raised body temperature and medical aid should be sought immediately.
Allergy to milk	A very small number of babies are allergic to cow's milk, and may produce symptoms if they are bottle fed. Commonly there is a history of asthma or eczema in either mother or father. The child produces a mild temperature with a blotchy rash and obvious colic. The best advice is to switch the feed from the formula used. There are special non-milk feed preparations based upon soya beans and vegetable proteins rather than those that come from an animal of a different species; these formulaes often help such a child. Medical advice is required and antihistamines may be needed.
Jaundice	Many babies appear yellow on the second to fifth day after birth. This is due to the normal process of breakdown of the baby's red blood cells. In the uterus, at a lower oxygen concentration, there were many more of these cells; once the baby is born, he is air-breathing and not so many red blood cells are needed, so they are disposed of. However, the liver of a newborn child is not very efficient in dealing with the breakdown products of haemoglobin, the iron pigment that carries the oxygen, and so an excess of yellow pigments spill over into the blood, temporarily showing as jaundice in the skin. Usually this is not serious but your doctor should be consulted. Blood tests may be necessary and the jaundice usually fades spontaneously; if it does not the doctor may suggest light treatment to the skin to help it go. In a very small number of cases the jaundice is due to a more serious problem, such as blockage of the bile ducts, or is a manifestation of a more generalized infection. Probably a fifth of babies become slightly jaundiced; this has no effect on their future life.

CIRCUMCISION

In the UK circumcision is not often performed; less than 6 per cent of newborn babies have the operation. If you wish this to be done, talk to your obstetrician before delivery so that should you have a male child, you and he are prepared. If the baby has to have circumcision then it is sensible to do it in the newborn period; if you leave it until the child is older, he will require a general anaesthetic and the whole procedure will be more serious. The operation on the newborn does not need a general anaesthetic. The foreskin is separated from the crown of the penis underneath and a plastic ring is passed around the whole organ. The skin is then removed and the ring, with a little silk suture on it, stops any bleeding.

Circumcision

The old rite of circumcision of the male newborn is still performed in some societies. If it is a part of your religious faith then it must be done, otherwise it is a completely unnecessary operation and can lead to problems of bleeding or infection. It is becoming rare now in the West, although some fathers feel that, having been circumcised themselves in their childhood, their male children should follow them. If it must be done, arrange for the operation in the first few days of life when it will affect the baby least.

The very small baby

Some babies are born small because they have been born before their time; others may be small in relation to the length of time they have been in the uterus. These babies used to be called premature, but are now more correctly called babies of low birthweight. They need special attention in the early days. If you are expected to have a baby like this you should deliver in a place that has the best possible pediatric services. The pediatrician who looks after the newborn child will be available at delivery and immediately afterwards with his full back-up team.

Babies who weigh between 2 and 2.5 kg are really very little different from their heavier brothers and sisters, but at weights below 2 kg a number of problems are likely to arise. Because the resistance to infection is lower, the baby will usually be isolated in a special unit. Here the staff are well aware of the problems of infection; they wear special clothes and take special precautions against this. There may be difficulty in maintaining respiration, so the small baby might require oxygen. This is usually by means of a head box

In the Special Care Unit a larger number of nurses are concentrated to give extra care to the very small immature babies. Such attention can only be given in large hospitals.

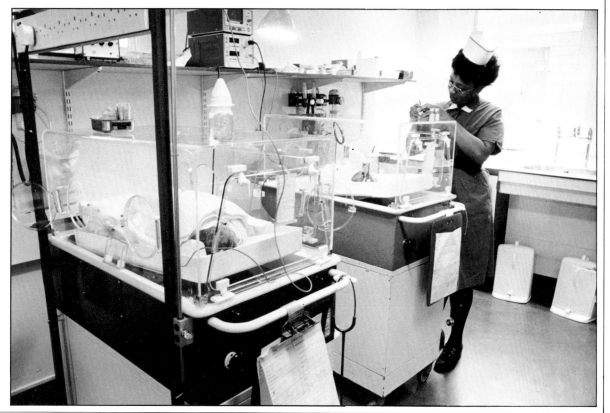

and incubator though it may mean the temporary passage of a tube into the air passages. The smaller the baby, the more difficult it is to maintain body temperature and this is helped by keeping him in an incubator. Many units used to nurse the baby without any clothes in order to observe the baby, but usually they now have some covering, either a light blanket or small baby clothing. Some immature infants are so small that ordinary baby clothing is too large. A special range of mini-clothes is made and sold in special shops — in difficulty, clothes made for dolls can be used.

Feeding may be difficult at first and the infant may require frequent small and dilute feeds. Sometimes he is tube-fed with expressed breast milk to help bypass the stage of swallowing. This is less alarming than it may sound and, in fact, the modern Special Care Baby Unit is run along very relaxed lines. Mother, father and other members of the family are encouraged to join in and help look after the baby.

Some people worry about the subsequent life of babies who were of low birthweight, but research has shown that low birthweight does not seem to interfere with the normal physical or mental course of development. Usually any low-birthweight infants who are going to be mentally or physically retarded show this in the first months of life; once the first year is passed, the unaffected infant may be considered as normal as his heavier brothers and sisters. Progress of the very low-birthweight infant to adult life has also been followed and it has been shown that normal children will grow into normal adults. When looking at Winston Churchill in his later years, it was hard to remember that he was a very low birthweight when he started. His later life showed no signs of his small beginning.

PERINATAL DEATH

Out of 50 women who attend the antenatal clinic, 49 will produce a live baby. However, one will have a baby who dies either in the last weeks of pregnancy or the first week after delivery. It is of little consolation to her that the numbers of perinatal deaths have been dropping, that the figure was 10 times this at the beginning of the century; statistics are meaningless where individual loss is concerned. The best way to guard against all risks in pregnancy is to get good care in the antenatal period and at the time of delivery. This usually means being under the care of a professional team of doctors and midwives who will try to prevent problems getting out of control by intercepting them at a very early stage. Their advice, based upon having seen many thousands of successful pregnancies and deliveries, is given specifically in order to prevent problems of illness and death in the perinatal period.

Stillbirth

A baby who dies before being born is called a stillbirth. He usually has been cut off from the oxygen supply in his mother's blood by some problem at the placenta or placental bed. We know of the obvious ones like separation of the placenta (see pages 92 to 93) where a clot of blood appears between the maternal and fetal blood circulations. Less obvious is when the blood supply from the mother's uterine arteries to the placental bed is diminished because of a narrowing inbuilt into the supplying blood vessels. This is associated with severe degrees of states such as pre-eclampsia and diabetes and it is for this that professionals watch so carefully in later pregnancy.

STILLBIRTH
In the rare but tragic event of a stillbirth, there is little that anyone can say or do to comfort the parents. It is important that they should be able to grieve fully so that eventually they can learn to live with the loss and perhaps try again for another baby. Many counsellors now feel that a good way to do this is to have a picture taken of the baby so that there is something permanent to remember him by. This may seem strange or even callous at the time, but most parents who have done this have been glad that they took the opportunity.

The parents of a newborn baby who is in danger of dying may wish to have him christened; most hospitals have the services of the clergy.

Premature birth

Babies who are born alive only to die soon afterwards are often suffering from the effects of immaturity. The smaller a baby is at birth, the more difficult it is to sustain life. Even so the pediatricians and their back-up teams have made the great advances in this area over the last few years. In a well-staffed pediatric intensive care unit, a baby born at 28 weeks now has approximately a 50 per cent chance of survival. Such a figure would have been impossible 10 years ago.

Serious abnormalities

Some children are born with congenital abnormalities (see Chapter 4) which are incompatible with life. Sad though it is that the baby dies, it is often thought by many couples to be better than a continued life with a major abnormality.

Oxygen starvation

A small number of babies suffer lack of oxygen during labour and, although born alive, die soon afterwards. Such oxygen starvation is watched for very carefully in labour and it is one of the major tasks of the professionals to try to predict it. It is not always apparent but often warning signs can be detected and action taken in time to prevent serious effects.

Rhesus disease and injuries

A major cause of death used to be rhesus disease but this has been overcome now by preventative measures (see pages 75 to 77). Similarly, injuries sustained at birth have been greatly reduced in numbers thanks to better training of doctors and midwives and better availability of their skills for all women having babies.

All the rationalizing that one can do about the loss of a baby becomes totally inadequate in the face of the human grief that the mother and father must feel in going home without their baby. The professionals will do all they can to soften the blow for they too are human beings, often with children of their own. Many parents get comfort from talking with other parents who have suffered similar catastrophes, who have realized that such problems are not necessarily recurrent and that family life can go on despite the catastrophe. Parents with similar bereavements can be contacted through the Stillbirth and Perinatal Death Association.

It is sad, but necessary, that a book about pregnancy and birth should also have to deal with perinatal death. Yet the miracle is that in slightly more than a century, the incidence of perinatal death has been reduced from a commonplace to a very rare event. I hope that these remarks on the subject of death will be of assistance to women who are concerned during pregnancy about the future health of their baby. I can only assure them that the vast majority of babies do not come into this category.

IS THE BABY NORMAL?

Every woman in pregnancy wonders if her child is normal and many women have fears of some malformation. This is a major concern and it is quite usual behaviour to worry about this. Fortunately, 98 per cent of babies born are quite normal, so that 49 out of 50 babies are not concerned in this section. The fact remains that 1 in 50 babies will face problems ranging from the most minor to the most serious. In this section, therefore, we will deal with some of the more common abnormalities. While the likelihood of their happening to any individual couple is small, I will discuss in more detail those who may be at increased risk for such a problem.

Less serious problems

The majority of abnormalities that occur in babies are not serious for either they correct themselves or they can be treated by some simple procedures in early life. Occasionally, a child is born with a small tag of skin in front of the ear. This is an extra auricle and is a reminder of the way the skin folds blended together in early fetal life. Such a skin tag is not serious; it has no effect on the child's hearing and, if it is worrying to the mother, may be removed by being tied off quite painlessly.

Extra digit

An extra digit may occasionally occur on the hands, or more uncommonly on the feet. It is usually without the full muscular and bony support of a conventional finger or toe and may be removed without a major operation.

Birth marks

Birth marks are sometimes found on the skin. Most are small red or blue marks, commonly on the trunk and particularly in the lower part. They are not caused by bruising but are minor variations in the small blood vessels of the skin. Most birth marks get smaller as the child grows. If treatment is required it is usually fairly simple, but a few of the larger birth marks, particularly those on the upper part of the body, will later require plastic surgical treatment; these are very much in the minority.

Talipes

Occasionally inside the uterus a fetus has localized pressure on his ankles and feet which leads to a turning in or, much more rarely, turning out of the foot at the ankle. This used to be called a club foot; the worse degrees are now very rarely seen. Often talipes is associated with a lack of amniotic fluid around the baby so that the ankle joints have been too cramped against the uterine wall. When a baby is born with a condition of talipes it is usually diagnosed very soon and the vast majority of such conditions can be coped with by a combination of exercises, massage and holding the ankle joint in special splints. The physiotherapist will begin in the hospital and will then teach the mother to do them in the home.

Dislocated hip

The hips of a child may not fit as tightly as do those of an adult and in consequence they may click when tested. This is the lowest grade of a possible dislocation and is always checked after birth. It can be treated by simple physiotherapy treatment and does not lead to permanent disability

Hernia

A hernia may occur at a weak spot in the muscles of the baby's stomach wall, allowing a part of the intestinal contents to bulge. This may be around the navel; usually this cures itself as the muscles strengthen after birth. It does not require taping or external support.

Undescended testes

The testicles are usually at the bottom of the scrotal sac when the child is born. Occasionally, however, they are not yet descended. This is not a serious matter for they may be situated at the upper part of the bag in the groin.

Hypospadias

A very small number of male children have the opening of the penis not at the tip but back along towards the shaft. This is not serious but may be a nuisance in later life when directing micturition. The problem is due to inexact fusion of the skin tube that makes up the penis and is not necesarily associated with more serious problems in the body.

None of these problems seriously threatens the future life and happiness of the child. However, they are a worry to parents and if they are detected they should be discussed fully with a paediatrician.

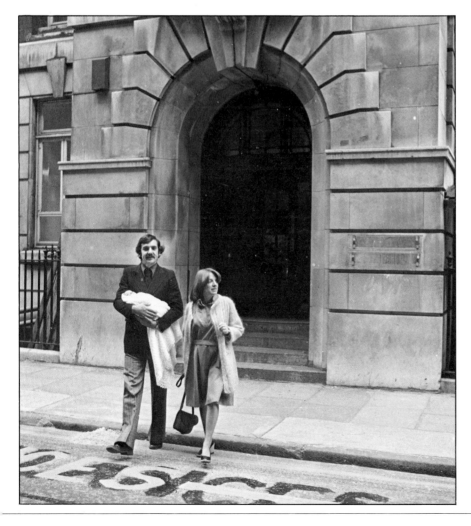

Going home to the start of a new family life.

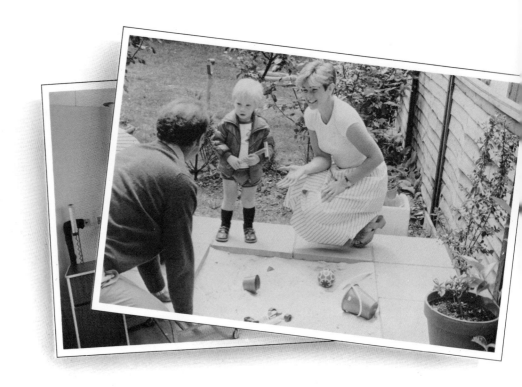

CONTRACEPTION

One of the most important aspects of bringing up a family is planning to have your children at intervals which suit you. Most couples now have the capacity to have children when they wish to, and not in a haphazard way. The sensible use of contraception should not be considered a negative aspect of life but a positive one which allows the couple to organize their chidren according to their economic and domestic commitments. One could add the freedom from unwanted childbirth to the other four basic freedoms, of speech, to worship, from want and from fear, laid down by Franklin D Roosevelt at the United Nations in its opening meeting in 1945. In large parts of the world contraception is probably the major advance to be made in establishing proper health care. In this section, however, we are not considering world population control but the individual planning of the family by the individual couple.

Ideally contraception should prevent pregnancy occurring while allowing intercourse to continue as normally as possible. It should be temporary and reversible at the wish of the couple using it. Unfortunately there is no ideal contraceptive agent; all have some inconvenience or side effects. Sterilization, a permanent barrier preventing sperm and the egg getting together, is not strictly a contraceptive method. However, I include it at the end of this section because more couples are now turning to sterilization once they think their family is complete.

HOW TO GET ADVICE

When considering which method of contraception might suit you, the whole range should be assessed. Different methods suit different couples and the same method may not suit you throughout your reproductive life. Pregnancy is not prevented by having intercourse in certain positions or by washing afterwards. Indeed, pregnancy can occur even if full penetration of the vagina by the penis has not taken place. Good contraceptive advice is best obtained in the UK from either your family doctor or a family planning clinic. Not all GPs give advice but if yours does not, you will be advised of another in the same district who does. Some women prefer the anonymity of the family planning clinic where you will see doctors and nurses especially trained in family planning methods. All professional advice is free; all appliances and drugs obtained at the clinic or from your GP are free to those entitled to the National Health Service. You may, if you prefer buy condoms from the chemist, but all other contraceptive devices need to be prescribed by your doctor.

HOW EFFECTIVE ARE THE METHODS?

All couples want to know the effectiveness of the method they are using. How likely is it to stop pregnancy? No method is 100 per cent perfect, not even sterilization. All have failure rates owing to the method being incorrectly used or the body reacting to the method in an unusual way. The simplest measure of efficiency is to consider the number of women out of 100 couples using the method for a year who get pregnant. This figure is usually expressed as the number of pregnancies per 100 woman years — 'hwy' for short. A very good method has a low rate, eg the pill is 0.3 per hwy; a less effective method would have a failure rate of 5 to 10 per hwy. Unguarded intercourse does not have a rate of 100 per hwy but nearer 60 to 70 per hwy.

METHODS USED BY BOTH PARTNERS

Rhythm method

This method of contraception depends upon not having intercourse at the time of ovulation. It is a good method if ovulation is regular. Most women make an egg about once every 28 days; if the egg is not fertilized, the lining of the uterus which was prepared to receive it is shed with vaginal bleeding some 14 days after egg production. This is a constant interval to within a day or two in all women. Thus, if you ovulate every 28 days you will probably menstruate every 28 days and egg production will fall almost precisely in the middle of the cycle. Should, however, your egg production be less frequent, say every 35 days, then the constant of 14 days from egg-making to menstruation still applies and so the first half of the cycle will be longer (21 days). It is essential to any one who wants to plan their conceptions using the rhythm method to understand this simple piece of biology. The timing of ovulation can be made precise by using one of several methods.

Basal temperature charts Take your temperature every morning before leaving bed and before smoking a cigarette or taking a cup of tea. After a month you will have a series of points on the chart. In the normal woman, these show a sustained rise in the second half of menstruation after egg-making has occurred. This is due to the release of the progesterone which causes all the body muscles to work a little harder and so drives the temperature up a little in the second half of the cycle. To check, the chart should be kept for two months.

Ovulation pain A few women actually know when they are ovulating; they sense a dull ache as the egg leaves the ovary. This mild discomfort is felt low in the pelvis, sometimes specific to one side or the other, but more often is poorly localized. A little fluid is released with the egg and this irritates the lining of the stomach cavity; the ache lasts for a few hours and is sometimes referred to by the German name — Mittelschmerz.

Cervical mucus The cervix is lined by cells that make mucus; these provide protection to the uterus and prevent the bacteria, normally present in the vagina, from rising higher into the uterus. For most of the menstrual cycle, the cervical mucus is thick and tacky but, within hours of egg-making, it becomes thin and slippery. The distinction between these two states can be appreciated by most women. If you slip a finger into the vagina in the morning and then rub that finger against your thumb you will find that for most of the time you can only separate the two digits by a centimetre or so before the string of mucus snaps. At the time of egg-making, however, you can stretch the mucus by as much as 6 cm as it has a lower surface tension than at other times.

The rhythm method is useful for it requires no medical intervention and costs nothing. However, it is wise to discuss details at your family planning clinic or with your doctor to make sure you have the timing right for your individual cycle. Rhythm is also an acceptable method to many whose faith prevents the use of other forms of contraception. The failure rate depends very much upon the effort the couple makes in trying to make it work. If a woman

The rhythm method depends on knowing when you are ovulating, and avoiding intercourse at that time.

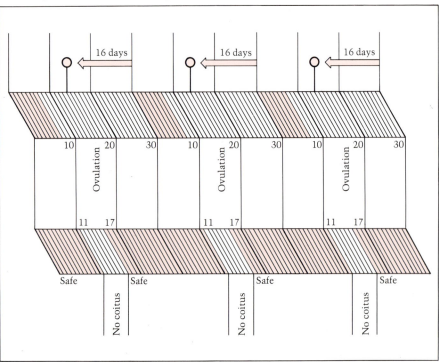

has irregular ovulation, she needs even more checks so that she actually knows her time of egg-making. The other major reason for failure of this method is that human beings are sometimes impatient and will not wait for the safe period. Consequently the failure rate varies from less than 2 to more than 15 per 100 woman years.

Incomplete intercourse

The term covers a number of extremely inefficient methods of contraception, which are nevertheless widely practised. Coitus interruptus occurs when the man removes his penis before ejaculation. Coitus reservatus is where, after introducing his penis into the vagina, he restricts his movements so much that no ejaculation occurs. Coitus interfemura takes places when he places his penis between the woman's legs so that there is no vaginal entry. These methods are often considered unsatisfactory by most couples, and quite understandably so. They impose a lot of responsibility on the man when he is usually not feeling very responsible and would prefer greater pleasure; in consequence they have a high failure rate. They are used very frequently for casual intercourse but the failure rate of up to 30 per 100 woman years makes them unacceptable when giving professional advice. As well as the danger of late withdrawal, sperm can escape from the penis before the main ejaculation of semen and these may be responsible for fertilization. Furthermore, even though semen is not deposited in the vagina, sperm from the outer lips of the entrance of the vagina can travel into the vagina and onwards.

METHODS BY THE MALE

Sheath

Although it may sound old fashioned, the sheath is the most common method of contraception used by married couples in the West. Sheaths are usually made of very thin latex. They come coated with a thin film of spermicidal jelly and are widely available in many outlets other than doctors' surgeries or family planning clinics. Some men think that the presence of a sheath interferes with sensation or impairs erection. Others object to the cost of the sheath — but this is, after all, very low. A very small number of men may have a localized chemical reaction on their penis either to the latex or the spermicidal cream.

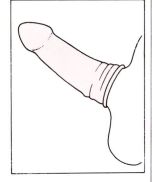

The common fear is that the sheath will rupture during intercourse, but this is a very rare event for each is tested extensively in the factories. However, the sheath may come off in the vagina if it is not pulled on properly over the full length of the erect penis, or if the man allows himself to stay in the vagina for too long after the erection has gone and the penis has become smaller and softer. The disadvantage of the sheath is that the man (or woman) must think and plan beforehand and have some available at the time of intercourse. The failure rates of 3 per hwy have been reported. With constant users this may drop below one.

The sheath is the most popular method of contraception used by married couples in this country. It must, however, be put on before there is any genital contact.

The male pill

There is not yet any safe and reliable form of male oral contraceptive. Many chemicals have been tried for their effect on sperm and have had good results in stopping sperm being made. However, as we noted earlier, one of the prime features of contraception is that it should be reversible. Most of the spermicidal agents tried so far are irreversible or have serious side effects.

METHODS USED BY THE FEMALE

Intravaginal chemicals and douches

There are many chemicals that kill sperm which are sold for use at the time of intercourse. They come in creams, pessaries, jellies and foams. All will greatly reduce the number of sperm provided they are put in the right place (the top of the vagina) at the right time (before intercourse starts). They only deal with one ejaculation at a time and must be repeated if multiple intercourse is going to occur. They are easy to buy and are cheap. Obviously a supply must be available at the time of intercourse, which may not be at the time the shops are open, so preparation is required. The most common cause of failure is that they are not put high enough into the vagina and failure rates of up to 20 per hwy are reported.

Douching is intended to wash away sperm after intercourse has occurred. It is often performed too late, for the most active sperm may be up the cervical canal out of reach of the douch before intercourse really finishes. The most frequently used douches contain a little acid (vinegar or lemon juice) and require some preparation: they must be used very soon after intercourse to be of any use and the failure rate is unacceptably high.

Vaginal diaphragms

These are thin circular rubber barriers on a spring ring which fit snugly between the top of the pubic bone and the back of the vagina. They come in different sizes and need medical help at the time of fitting. They must be of the correct size to be both effective and comfortable. The vaginal diaphragm must be put in before each intercourse and not removed until six to eight hours afterwards to allow for the few sperm that stay active longer than the rest. It is best used in conjunction with a spermicidal cream in case any sperm manage to get around the edge.

Some women find diaphragms a nuisance: either they must be put in every night or else just before intercourse is about to occur, and this may interfere with the emotions of that particular occasion. The failure rate of a vaginal diaphragm used properly is low, in the order of 2 per hwy. Very rarely, they may get misplaced at the time of intercourse; in some women the pelvic muscles change after a pregnancy or alteration of weight so the diaphragm no longer fits properly. This should be checked.

The soft, thin rubber diaphragm fits snugly into the vagina, with the rubber-covered spring at the edge holding snugly to the walls. It is easily inserted, but you will need some help from the family planning clinic or your doctor the first time you do it.

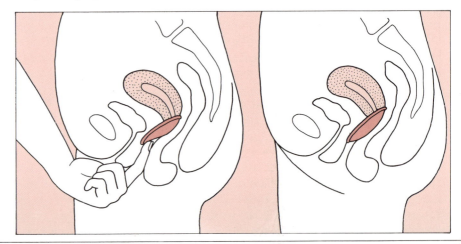

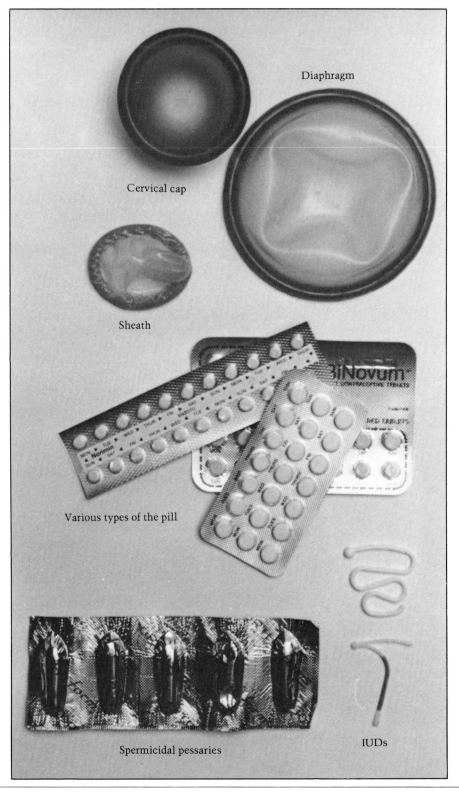

Diaphragm

Cervical cap

Sheath

Various types of the pill

Spermicidal pessaries

IUDs

Contraceptives work in a variety of ways: these include preventing sperms reaching the egg by barrier methods (diaphragm, cervical cap and sheath); killing sperm before they can reach the egg (spermicidal creams and pessaries); preventing the ovaries releasing the egg or preventing its implantation (the pill and IUDs).

Cervical cap

This is a small thick-walled rubber dome fitting accurately over the cervix itself. It is used in conjunction with spermicidal jelly. You will need medical help to get the correct size and the size must be checked after each pregnancy. It must be put in before intercourse and left in place for six to eight hours afterwards; more spermicidal jelly is required for a repeated intercourse. However, inserting the cap requires even more knowledge and awareness of the tissues of the pelvis by the woman than does the diaphragm, and may call for more patience to fit. The failure rate is about the same as that of the vaginal diaphragm.

The cervical cap is a thick rubber dome fitting over the cervix. It must be inserted correctly so that it adheres to the surface of the cervix.

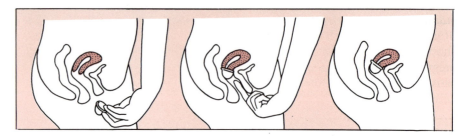

Intrauterine contraceptive device (IUD)

This is a foreign body made of plastic (or plastic coated with metal) which rests permanently in the uterine cavity to prevent a pregnancy. IUDs can all be straightened out for insertion into the uterus and they then take up their position fitting snugly inside the cavity. They can usually be put in by a doctor without any anaesthetic, particularly if a woman has had a baby before, and once inserted no action need be taken at the time of intercourse. This is a major advantage. A fine nylon tail is usually left through the neck of the womb into the vagina so that the woman can check for herself that the IUD is still in place and has not been moved, particularly during a menstrual period.

The precise mode of action of the IUD is not known but probably the surface area irritates the lining of the uterus so that no egg can settle there. In addition, it may, by reflex action, interfere with the muscles of the Fallopian tubes and so sperm travelling up the tube to meet an egg have greater difficulty. Those loops with a metallic coating may also have a chemical action on sperm while they are passing up the uterine cavity.

About 10 per cent of women who have an intrauterine device have heavier

An IUD is inserted in the uterus by a doctor or trained nurse. They check the length of the body of the uterus first and then insert the device in a straightened out form (*far right*). Once inside the uterus, the outer sheath is removed and the coil resumes its normal shape (*right*).

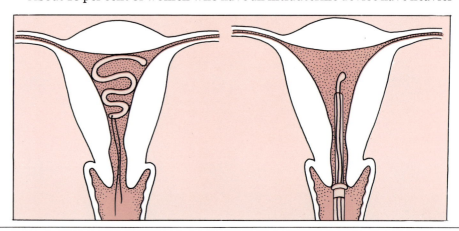

periods afterwards. It is difficult to tell which women will fall into this group, so if you think an IUD is the best method of contraception, try it and see; it can always be removed fairly easily. A proportion of women who have heavy periods afterwards do so for three or four cycles only and then return to normal. A few women get a vaginal discharge from irritation by the nylon tail in the cervical canal. Sometimes a pre-existing infection of the pelvis is flared up by the presence of this foreign body. Very rarely, the device can migrate into the wall of the uterus and so be ineffective.

The intrauterine devices have a very low failure rate of 0.5 to 2 per hwy. Most failures are due to explusion at the time of menstruation, but a very small number of women can get pregnant despite a properly retained intra-uterine device. If this happens, the device can be removed in early pregnancy; should the woman not realize until she is more than about three months pregnant, most obstetricians would leave the intrauterine device in place. It causes no harm to the baby and usually comes away with the placenta after delivery.

Oral contraception (The pill)

The pill is a hormone tablet taken each day to prevent egg-making. It is probably the most popular method of contraception among young married couples in the West. It is still relatively new so that, when any of the rare complications occur, they are widely reported. Most oral contraceptives are an oestrogen-progestogen mixture and are taken from the fifth to twenty-fifth day of the menstrual cycle. During the rest of the cycle when no pill is taken bleeding occurs caused by withdrawal of the oestrogen; strictly speaking this should not be called a period for no egg has been made. Contraception probably suppresses egg-making by interfering with the hormones produced from the pituitary gland. There is probably an additional effect on the cervical mucus so that it is not thinned out in the middle of the cycle and sperm therefore have difficulty in getting to the uterus.

Some pills contain progestogen only. These are particularly useful at the time of breast feeding or if a woman cannot take oestrogens. They are not quite so effective as the combined pills but they still give good contraceptive action. Egg-making probably still occurs; the mini pill acts on the cervical mucus and possibly interferes in addition with the transport of sperm and eggs in the Fallopian tube. Some oral contraceptives contain a sequential dose of oestrogens for 14 days followed by an oestrogen-progestogen mixture for 7 days. These are useful if a woman experiences side effects from the regular pill.

ORAL CONTRACEPTION AND CANCER OF THE CERVIX
One of the fears of those who take oral contraceptives is that the altered hormone background may increase the risks of cancer. Recent research has further raised fears of a link between cancer of the cervix and breast and use of oral contraception. The research actually linked the risk to those who started taking the pill very early in life, and this was a risk already known to the medical profession for many years. Unfortunately, the research was reported out of context and raised many unnecessary fears. Be very careful not to be scared into stopping the pill by ill-judged and usually ill-informed newspaper comments.

The pill probably works by interfering with ovulation. It is taken by mouth and absorbed from the intestinal tract; after being metabolized in the liver it is passed into the bloodstream. Some chemicals move to the pituitary gland in the brain. There they interfere with the hormones which normally travel down to the ovary to stimulate ovulation. Thus the pill, although it also affects the hormone secretions which cause the cervix to become ripe also probably works by interfering with ovulation.

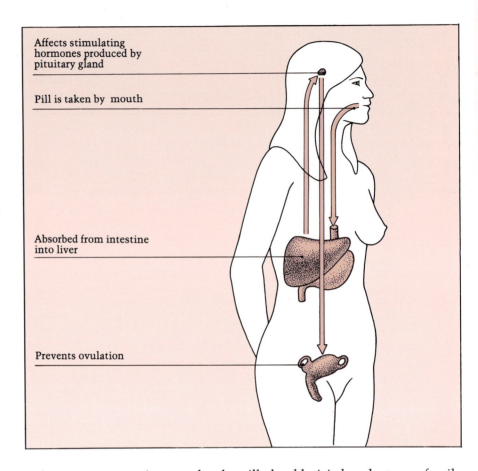

Affects stimulating hormones produced by pituitary gland

Pill is taken by mouth

Absorbed from intestine into liver

Prevents ovulation

Any woman wanting to take the pill should visit her doctor or family planning clinic. They will check her health and start her on a low-dosage pill of proven efficacy. There are many of these on the market and most are now packaged in useful aide memoire containers with a monthly supply of pills in each, so that you can see whether you have taken the appropriate pill for the day. One of the major reasons for failure of oral contraception is simply forgetting to take a pill, especially in the middle of the month. It is found that the pill is not such a safe method among those who are not regular in their habits. The packet of pills should be kept somewhere where you do a regular daily event such as cleaning your teeth or making coffee in the morning. The doctor who prescribes the pill will probably want to see you again after a few months to make sure that the pill suits you. For the majority, the first pill prescribed suits and can be taken for as long as required, subject to a short, yearly check by GP or family planning clinic. If there are no problems, the pill can be used for many years until the age of 38 or 40.

Problems can occur with nausea or with weight gain. These can be helped by altering the pill to provide a different oestrogen dosage. Some women have breakthrough bleeds — spotting of blood at the wrong days of the cycle. This again can be helped by a lower dose of one of the two components of the pill. As well as the nuisance side effects there are some serious side effects which receive much publicity. The most important is the increased risk of clot formation in the blood vessels. The blood of women on the pill is slightly altered in its chemical constitution and there is therefore a slight tendency to clotting. This is not a serious risk in younger women but for those over the age of 40 the risk rate increases.

Much publicity is given to the relationship of the pill and cancer. Oral contraception only started in the late 1950s and we have not got enough accumulated information to give a certain answer. The probability is, however, that the lower-dose pills now used by most women do not have any effect of increasing cancer rate of any organ; they may even act as a protective agent to protect you against certain growths such as cancer of the lining of the uterus and the ovary. Any scientific research quoted in the newspapers and on television needs careful interpretation. Often headlines are made of one minute part of the research and the balancing comments elsewhere are not mentioned. If there are scares about the pill ask someone who can assess all the evidence in the latest research. Best advice comes from your professionals; if you have any doubts about your pill discuss it freely with your GP or family planning clinic before thinking of stopping it. The actual risks of being pregnant unwantedly might be greater than the theoretical ones of longer-term malignancy.

The failure rates of the pill are very low, about 0.1 to 0.5 per hwy. As we have mentioned, the most common reason for failure is forgetting to take the pill — although a small number of women have a breakthrough of pituitary hormone to cause an egg to be produced. This is exceedingly rare, as the figures suggest.

The morning-after pill

Occasionally there may be unguarded intercourse unexpectedly in the middle of the cycle. It is too late to turn to conventional contraception and so a method has been evolved to try to stop the fertilized egg from implanting. A high dose of oestrogen taken in the first day as the egg is travelling down the tube can prevent implantation. This is not recommended as a regular means of contraception but, should the problem arise, you should visit your family doctor or clinic within 24 hours of the event. They will provide you with several pills to be taken by mouth. Unfortunately, this high oestrogen dosage may cause nausea, but many women will be prepared to put up with that to avoid the inconvenience of a completely unwanted pregnancy.

STERILIZATION

As stressed previously, sterilization should not be considered as a method of contraception for it is not reversible. Today, however, many couples are turning to sterilization once they feel their family is complete. Sterilizing operations may be performed on the male or female.

Male sterilization

Sperm is carried from the testis, where it is made, to the storage sac behind the prostate gland. At a male sterilization this tube is divided in the groin near the top of the scrotal sac. The operation is a vasectomy. It can be done under local anaesthetic each side and takes about 20 minutes. It is a minor procedure and the man can usually return to his normal activities a day or so later. Since some sperm has already passed the point of division at the operation and is being stored in the storage sac, it may take a few months before these are all

The tube conveying sperm from the testis is isolated in the groin. In a vasectomy it is divided and the ends turned back to stop it rejoining.

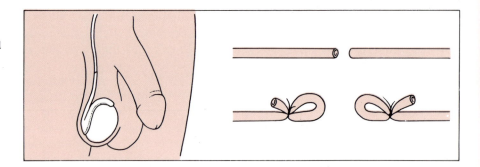

used up at intercourse. In consequence, contraception must be continued along conventional lines for at least three months until all the sperm in the pipeline have been expelled. This is usually checked by semen analysis monthly and unguarded intercourse should only take place after two successive samples show no sperm. Obviously the more often the man has intercourse (using conventional contraception) in this time, the quicker he will flush out the sperm already in the system.

This is a small operation and a much lesser procedure than the female sterlization but it seems to carry greater psychological overtones. Men fear the loss of their masculinity after vasectomy, although this is completely unfounded. There is no change of sexual feelings or performance after the operation. Men still make the same volume of seminal fluid, for this comes from the prostate gland; it just does not have any sperm in it. They will go on performing as well (or as badly) as they did before and fears about loss of libido need not be considered.

Female sterilization

Female sterilization is carried out by sealing the Fallopian tubes, which go from the ovary to the uterus. This involves a formal operation, opening the stomach, usually under a general anaesthetic, and therefore a stay in hospital. The operation can be performed through a small incision in the stomach or by inserting a laparoscope into an incision on the lower part of the navel. The Fallopian tubes can be cut and turned back so that they cannot rejoin; through the laparoscope, the tubes may be cauterized to destroy a 2 cm length or they may be clipped or banded. The exact method of sterilization will depend upon your body size and shape and the surgeon performing it. Discuss this fully with him beforehand. Usually there are no serious after effects to sterilization although a few women have heavier periods for some time afterwards. Sex life will remain the same and there will be no alteration in your sexual performance.

It must be stressed that neither male nor female sterilization is perfect. There is a small failure rate for each in the order of 2 to 4 times per 1,000 operations performed. This means that 996 to 998 couples per 1,000 of those sterilized will be perfectly safe. The most common reason for failure is not that the operation has not been done properly but that the tissues have regenerated or that the mechanical clip or ring has not done its job perfectly. Most surgeons who perform sterilization operations will warn you of this and the majority would be willing to see anyone who had a failure of sterilization afterwards to help them cope with the problem.

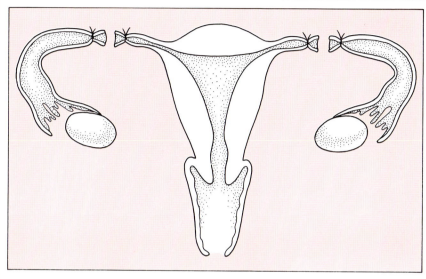

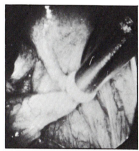
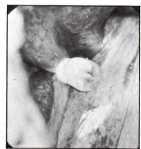

Each Fallopian tube is divided so that the sperm rising from the vagina cannot meet the egg coming from the ovary. This may be done by cutting (*above*), by cauterization (*far left*) or by closing the tube with an elastic band (*left*).

FUTURE ADVANCES IN CONTRACEPTION

In many areas of the world knowledge about the availability and benefits of contraception needs to be greatly expanded. This is the most important advance that can happen. In the West research will continue, probaby in the area of the male pill, although there is no sign of a breakthrough yet. It is unlikely that in the next decade many further changes in the female pill will happen. Research is proceeding into the production of antibodies which would act against sperm and so prevent conception. There is also research into the effect that pituitary hormones have in initiation of the cycle which leads to egg-making.

Methods of local contraception are being improved. The male sheath is now made of thinner rubber without loss of strength and so provides better sensation. Vaginal caps and preparations are being refined; sponges and rings impregnated with hormones or spermicidal chemicals are being tested. Experiments are taking place with reversible methods of sterilization by which the tubes carrying the sperm or the egg may be temporarily closed by a plug or valve which can be removed later. However, the greatest advance in family planning in the next decade will be a wider acceptance and use of the methods we have already pioneered, so that they can be properly applied and not left on the chemist's shelves or in the drawers of bed-side cabinets.

GLOSSARY

During the course of your antenatal care your will hear doctors and midwives use technical terms which may convey nothing to you. Many of these words have been used in the main text and have been explained in context. This is a ready reference section which lists the most frequently used technical terms together with a brief explanation of their meaning.

AFTERPAINS
Contractions of the uterus occur in the days and weeks after delivery as the last of the clots and fragments of tissue are expelled. These tightenings of the uterine muscle can be strong enough to make you use pain-relieving drugs.

ALPHA FETOPROTEIN
From the early days of pregnancy the fetus makes alpha fetoprotein and secretes it in the fluid of its nervous system. If there is a gap in the coverings of that nervous system, as happens in conditions such as anencephaly or spina bifida, then the alpha fetoprotein can leak from the fetus into the fluid which surrounds it and thus be absorbed by the mother. A raised level of alpha fetoprotein will then be found in her blood and this is taken as an indication that there may be a problem of the baby's spine or head.

AMNIOCENTESIS
Amniocentesis is the process by which fluid is removed from the baby's amniotic sac, through the mother's abdominal wall. It is a simple process and does not require a general anaesthetic. The fluid can be examined for alpha fetoprotein (q.v.) or for chromosome

changes such as Down's Syndrome (q.v.). Later in pregnancy, amniotic fluid may be used to check the maturity of the fetus or to assessing any problems in connection with rhesus incompatibility.

AMNIOTIC FLUID The baby lives surrounded by fluid, which is made from the amnion. The fluid acts as a packing material, buffering him from shocks and changes in temperature. He grows inside the fluid until just before birth when the membranes around him burst and the amniotic fluid leaks away.

ANALGESICS
Analgesics are pain-relieving drugs. Pain can be relieved by numbing the nerves or by dimming the sensations. An epidural anaesthetic (q.v.) blocks the nerves as they flow from the spine. Pethidine dims sensations and makes you less aware of what is going on. Inhalation analgesia (q.v.) also dims sensations.

BEARING DOWN The bearing-down sensation is the instinctive urge to push the baby out once the neck of the womb has opened. It is important to keep this urge under control and to push only as directed

by your midwife. You will be able to try this out in antenatal classes.

BRAXTON HICKS CONTRACTIONS
Contractions of the uterus start early in pregnancy but are not usually noticed by the mother until the last weeks. It is usual to feel some tightenings of the uterus from about 30 weeks. These contractions can at times become strong enough to make you hold your breath but they are most often not painful.

BREECH In the last weeks of pregnancy the baby takes up his final position in the uterus; this is mostly head downwards. However, approximately three per cent of babies present by the breech, i.e. bottom downwards. When this happens extra precautions must be taken by the obstetrician.

CATHETER A catheter is a thin, hollow plastic or rubber tube which may be used to release urine from the bladder.

CHORIONIC BIOPSY
Chorionic biopsy is a method of obtaining tissue from the growing embryo at a very early stage of pregnancy (about eight weeks). A suction cannula is passed up through the

vagina and the cervix; some fetal tissue is taken under ultrasound guidance. The tissue can then be used to examine chromosome patterns. If an abnormality is detected, termination of pregnancy may be recommended at about 11 or 12 weeks.

COLIC The intestinal muscle occasionally becomes overactive and tightens excessively on the contents (liquid or solid) inside the bowel. The sufferer, responds by feeling pain. An adult will know what is going on and understand, a baby cannot understand and responds by pulling up his legs, going puce and screaming.

COLOSTRUM The breasts do not produce milk immediately after delivery. Initially they produce colostrum — a clear fluid, low in fat, and high in nutritional value.

DILATATION The cervix holds the baby in place throughout pregnancy. During labour it has to open up from 0 to 10cm in a few hours. This process is called dilatation and once it is completed, the baby's head can pass down into the vagina and so be delivered.

DILATION AND CURETTAGE (D and C) Occasionally the doctor has to evacuate the contents of the uterus because of excessive bleeding after delivery; sometimes a pregnancy stops in the first weeks and the embryo is absorbed, but the lining of the womb has not come away. In both these instances, the cervix must be dilated gently under anaesthesia and a small curved instrument used to scrape away the lining of the womb and any products that may be inside the uterus. It is quite a common operation, which is done under general anaesthesia and does not hurt.

ECLAMPSIA Occasionally, a woman whose blood pressure is raised in pregnancy goes on to have a series of fits. This used to be a common and major cause of death. With good antenatal care and preventative medicine eclampsia has become very rare.

EFFACEMENT OF THE CERVIX The process by which, prior to dilation (q.v.), the cervix shortens and flattens into a ring of muscle.

ENGAGEMENT When the widest diameter of the baby's head passes through the brim of the mother's pelvis it is said to have engaged. This often happens in the last weeks of pregnancy and is a sign that the baby will probably be able to negotiate the rest of the pelvis and be born vaginally.

ENGORGEMENT OF BREASTS Once the baby is born, the breasts produce milk rapidly; if the baby does not take enough, the milk becomes static in the breasts, and they become engorged and stretched. At first the balance between production of milk and removal by the baby is not well organized; it takes a week or two for production and removal to balance. Ice packs or hot flannels may help to reduce the worst effects of engorgement.

ENTONOX Entonox is a mixture of equal parts of nitrous oxide and oxygen. It is a good means of pain relief for the later stages of labour.

EPIDURAL ANALGESIA One of the better ways of stopping pain in labour is to inject a local anaesthetic into the epidural space. This is outside the spinal cord and its coverings, where the nerves flow away to the organs including the uterus. An epidural analgesic requires a skilled anaesthetist. Most women who have had an epidural on one occasion will ask for one for a second.

EPISIOTOMY An episiotomy is a clean incision made in the tissues at the bottom of the vagina to ease the passage of the baby's head. This is usually done under local anaesthetic.

EXPRESSION OF BREAST MILK Milk may be removed from the breast by expression, either by hand or by means of a small breast pump. The milk may be put into a sterilized bottle and used for baby feeds when the mother is not available. Breast milk collected in this way may also be frozen for future use. Some women make more milk than their baby needs. If the excess is collected it can be used to feed the very small babies in Special Care Baby Units. Ask your local hospital if they need milk; the National Childbirth Trust also organizes milk collections.

EXTENSION OF THE HEAD The baby usually comes down the vaginal canal with his head well flexed and his chin tucked against his chest. Occasionally, the head is not well tucked in but is extended so that wider diameters have to negotiate the pelvis.

EXTERNAL ROTATION After delivery of the baby's head from the mother's vulva, the shoulders have to rotate into the long axis of the mother's pelvis. This means that the whole baby has to move through 90 degrees. From the outside the baby's head can be seen to rotate, so that instead of looking directly backwards, it turns to look towards one of the mother's thighs.

FACE PRESENTATION While most babies tuck their chin against their chest, so that the top of the head presents, occasionally the head is extended so much that the baby is looking straight down at the cervix and thus the face presents. This is usually diagnosed in labour and, provided care is taken, a vaginal delivery can occur.

FERTILIZATION When the ovum is penetrated by a sperm in the lateral end of the Fallopian tube, fertilization occurs.

FETAL DISTRESS In unusual cases the fetus can become short of oxygen in the uterus. This is shown by alterations in the heart beat and in the movements. These are watched for carefully in the last weeks of pregnancy and in labour.

FETAL MONITORING These are measurements made of the fetus in pregnancy and in labour. **During pregnancy** the fetus may be monitored by recording on a special chart the kicks the baby makes inside the uterus. In addition, fetal wellbeing can be assessed by checking the hormone and proteins made by the placenta. Further, the fetal heart rate can be examined in the antenatal clinic by cardiotography.

During labour, fetal monitoring concentrates on the fetal heart rate. If the fetal heart monitor shows signs of problems inside the uterus, a small sample of blood can be drawn from the baby by fetal blood scalp sampling and his exact oxygen state can be determined.

FETAL MOVEMENTS In the uterus, the fetus moves his arms and legs and wriggles his body. He also makes slower movements of the head and chest. Some of these movements start very early in pregnancy, but the mother does not notice them until about 16 to 20 weeks. They can be observed by ultrasound methods much earlier than this and they are a valuable sign of wellbeing. If the movements a baby makes are reduced, you should report this to your midwife or doctor; in most cases it means the baby is sleeping, but it could be a warning sign that there is some danger to the fetus.

FETUS (FOETUS) Fetus is the name generally given to the growing unborn child. After fertilization, the clump of cells is known as the blastocyst and then the morula. After this, organs start to form and the new individual is called an embryo. Once organogenesis has finished, by about 10 weeks, the term fetus is

used and this is the name for the unborn child until delivery.

FONTANELLES The fetal skull must allow rapid growth of the brain underneath, both before and after birth. In consequence, the junction to the various flat bones of the skull are not fused, but allow for stretch. At the points where the several junctions meet there is a membrane closing over the gap, this is called the fontanelle.

FUNDUS The fundus is the top of the uterus. Some obstetricians use this as a measure of the growth of the baby. The upper end of the uterus represents the upper end of growth, and its changing relationship with landmarks in the mother's abdomen shows that fetal growth is occurring.

HYPERTENSION Abnormally high blood pressure. Your blood pressure is checked at every antenatal visit to ensure that there is no departure from the normal range. Prompt action will be taken to control any such departures.

HYPOTENSION Abnormally low blood pressure.

INDUCTION Obstetricians sometimes recommend that labour should be started before nature does. Labour is induced when it is considered that the risks to the fetus of staying inside the uterus are

greater than the risks of being outside. In the United Kingdom about a quarter of all labours are induced, and the commonest reasons are pre-eclampsia (q.v.) and postmaturity (q.v.). Labour can be induced by the use of prostaglandin pessaries or by breaking the membranes.

INHALATION ANALGESIA If the pain-relieving methods are taken in through the lungs, they are said to be inhaled.

INVOLUTION After delivery, the uterus and other organs of the pelvis return to their non-pregnant state by involuting. This takes four or six weeks to happen.

LAPAROSCOPE Occasionally a doctor wishes to see inside the abdominal cavity without having to make a formal incision. This sometimes happens when a woman has abdominal pain in early pregnancy and it is thought that the pregnancy is outside the cavity of the uterus — an ectopic pregnancy. Under general anaesthesia, a laparoscope, a tube about 1cm in diameter, can be passed through a very small incision in the lower border of the umbilicus. The laparoscope carries a lens system and a light source so that the doctor can look carefully at the organs in the abdomen. Operations via

laparoscope are very limited and it is used mainly to make a diagnosis.

LIGHTENING In the last weeks of pregnancy, the fetus descends into the pelvis and the head engages (q.v.). In consequence, there is much less bulk in the upper part of the uterus and you will notice, with great relief, that your stomach and intestines can take up more space. The lightening effect may occur as early as 36 weeks in someone having their first baby, but usually a little later on with subsequent babies.

LOCHIA After the baby is born the uterus still has some excessive lining, and fragments of the membranes may remain. These are expelled with blood for the first few days after delivery. As time goes by the blood component fades, so the lochia become yellow and eventually white. They should stop by two or three weeks after a normal delivery, or by three or four weeks after a Caesarean section.

MEMBRANES These are elastic, stretchy substances which grow with the baby. When, at the end of pregnancy or in early labour, he no longer needs the membranes, they rupture just over the cervix and the amniotic fluid drains away. One of the ways of inducing labour (q.v.) is to rupture the membranes. This is called ARM — artificial rupture of the membranes.

MOULDING As the fetal head passes down through the bony pelvis, it has to negotiate the passages and the head becomes slightly altered in shape. Bones of the skull overlap each other and so the head is moulded into the shape of the mother's pelvis. A long labour produces more moulding than others; babies born by Caesarean section have virtually no moulding.

N.A.D. This abbreviation means Nothing Abnormal Detected. Most women will see this in their antenatal notes as they go through pregnancy with no problems.

OCCIPITO-ANTERIOR AND OCCIPITO-POSTERIOR The occiput is the back of the skull. It is used as a marker of the way in which the head is facing. An occipito-anterior position means that the back of the baby's head is towards the mother's front and he can flex his head well on to his chest and so is likely to pass through the pelvis more readily. When the presentation ia occiput-posterior, it is more difficult for him to flex his head for his spine is now against the mother's spine.

OEDEMA When the body retains salt, it also retains fluid, and this is reflected by swelling of the tissues. Many women suffer from oedema in pregnancy, particularly in warm weather. It occurs at the ankles, in the fingers, or in the face.

OESTROGENS One of the two major hormones produced in pregnancy is oestrogen. This is a steroid hormone produced, in the first instance, by the ovary and later by the placenta. It enables the uterus to get ready to receive the growing blastocyst and later to accommodate the fetus as he grows. It also helps to increase the blood supply to the uterus and so to the growing fetus. The breasts respond to oestrogen as do many other organs of the body.

OLIGOHYDRAMNIOS The amniotic fluid (q.v.) around the baby provides the packing material that allows him to grow in a fairly unrestrained fashion. Oligohydramnios means that there is a lack of fluid; the fetus may be confined inside the uterine sac and his growth restricted.

OXYTOCIN DRIP Oxytocin is the man-made equivalent of pitocin, the hormone which helps to start the uterus contracting. If the obstetrician thinks induction should occur he may start labour with oxytocin.

Occasionally, women who actually started spontaneously go rather slowly in mid-labour and so oxytocin is used intravenously. This is not induction of labour but acceleration of a normally started process.

PALPATION The obstetrician or midwife palpates the abdomen at each antenatal visit in order to check the growth of the uterus and, in later months, the growth of the fetus and his position.

PELVIC FLOOR The floor of the pelvis is made up of muscle which is pierced in three places, by the urethra carrying urine in front, the vagina in the middle, and the rectum carrying faeces at the back. The pelvic floor has to be strong enough to prevent the contents of the abdomen from slipping down. However, it must also be flexible enough to allow a baby to pass through at the end of pregnancy. Often, the stretch required by this process leads to weakness of the pelvic floor and prolapse may occur in later life. An episiotomy can relieve the muscles during labour and allow the baby to pass more readily.

PERINEUM The perineum refers to the tissues at the outlet of the vagina which may require division as in an episiotomy (q.v.).

PETHIDINE An analgesic drug which is used to relieve pain in labour. It is usually given by injection and produces a drowsy, non-caring state.

PITUITARY GLAND The pituitary gland is at the base of the skull and produces hormones that control egg-production and the action of the uterus. The pituitary gland stimulates egg-production and is, therefore, essential to getting a pregnancy started; once pregnancy has begun other hormones are produced which help the uterus to accommodate the growing fetus and the breasts to produce milk.

PLACENTA The placenta is the essential exchange station through which the fetus receives all the nutrients and oxygen which he needs during pregnancy. Once the baby is born it is usually delivered fairly easily in the third stage of labour. It is also known as the afterbirth.

POLYHYDRAMNIOS The baby is protected in the uterus by the amniotic fluid (q.v.) which surrounds him. On occasions excess fluid is made. The baby can then float around too freely and he may take up unusual positions, which make delivery difficult.

POSTMATURITY A postmature pregnancy is one which lasts more than 42 weeks from the first day of the last normal menstrual period. Most obstetricians feel that by 42 weeks it will be safer for both mother and baby if the baby is delivered and induction will be offered.

PRE-ECLAMPSIA Pre-eclampsia is a condition in pregnancy in which blood pressure is raised, there is protein in the urine and oedema (q.v.). In extreme cases it could lead to eclampsia (q.v.). Nowadays, antenatal care usually prevents the extreme occurring, but pre-eclampsia can still lead to a diminished supply of blood to the placental bed. If this happens the fetus will have a reduced supply of nutrients in pregnancy and oxygen during labour.

Careful monitoring is carried out in the last weeks of pregnancy to ensure that the blood pressure does not rise and that there is no protein in the urine.

PRETERM LABOUR A preterm labour is one which starts more than three weeks before the due date, i.e. before the 37th week of pregnancy. The earlier this is, the more likely it is to be associated with a baby who is immature and is not ready for the outside world. Preterm labours at 36 and 37 weeks are not serious but a baby

born at 30 weeks is very immature and will require very special care.

PROGESTERONE Progesterone is one of the major hormones made in the body during pregnancy. It is produced at first from the ovary and later by the placenta; it helps the uterus to accommodate the growing fetus, and the mother's body to adapt to the changes that occur in pregnancy.

PUERPERIUM This is the time of recovery after childbirth and the return to normal function of the organs. It usually lasts six weeks.

QUICKENING When a mother first feels fetal movement (q.v.) at about 16 to 20 weeks she has felt the baby quicken. Emotionally, this is a very important time, but it is not a helpful indication of the maturity of the pregnancy.

RIPENING OF THE CERVIX In the last weeks of pregnancy the cervix is said to ripen, it becomes softer, the canal is taken up and some dilatation occurs. Not all women start labour with a closed cervix and many, particularly those who have had a baby before, have some degree of dilatation and effacement of the cervix (q.v.) before labour starts.

Occasionally, induction of labour (q.v.) is considered

necessary, but the cervix is unripe. The cervix can be ripened by the insertion of prostaglandin pessaries into the upper vagina.

SECOND STAGE OF LABOUR Labour is divided into three stages; the second stage starts with full dilatation of the cervix and finishes with delivery of the baby. This is the most satisfying stage as you can push with contractions to help the baby's descent through the pelvis.

SHOW When the cervix is taken up at the beginning of labour, a plug of mucus (q.v.) is shed and comes out through the vagina. This is the mucus show. Sometimes, with the plug of mucus, there is a little bleeding from the surface vessels of the cervical canal; this is the bloody show. A show of mucus or blood is a sign of the imminence of labour.

SYNTOCINON The pituitary gland makes the hormone oxytocin which stimulates uterine contractions. Syntocinon is the man-made product has the same action and is used in induction of labour.

SYNTOMETRINE When the uterus contracts at the end of the third stage of labour, the placenta has been expelled and usually there is little bleeding. However, if the uterus does not contract firmly the

woman can bleed heavily and become very ill. Syntometrine is a drug given to all women at the end of delivery in order to make the uterus firm and prevent bleeding.

THIRD STAGE The third stage of labour starts with the delivery of the baby and finishes with the delivery of the placenta. It is a short stage lasting only a few minutes.

TRANSVERSE LIE Most babies settle in the uterus in a longitudinal position. They present therefore by the head or vertex (q.v.) or by the breech (q.v.). However, a small percentage of babies take up a horizontal position. If the baby does not move into a longitudinal position a Caesarean section will be necessary.

ULTRASOUND Ultrasound waves are very high frequency sound waves. Ultrasound can be used to check the size and growth of the baby. It is safe by conventional standards and, despite recent concern over its use, there is no evidence that it causes any harm to the mother or to the baby in subsequent life.

VERTEX The vertex is a rectangular area of the skull of the fetus which presents in well-flexed head presentations. If your midwife can feel this, it is a sign of good fetal progress.

INDEX